Obs and Gynae

PG Focus Series

Liver Disorders in Pregnancy

Obs and Gynae
PG Focus Series
Liver Disorders in Pregnancy

Editors

Komal N Chavan

MD DNB MNAMS FCPS DGO FICOG and Diploma in Reproductive Medicine (UK-SH Germany)
Senior Consultant and Unit Chief
Department of Obstetrics and Gynaecology
VN Desai Hospital
Mumbai, Maharashtra, India

Niranjan Chavan

MD FICOG FCPS DGO DFP MICOG DICOG Diploma in Endoscopy (USA)
Professor and Unit Chief
Department of Obstetrics and Gynaecology
Lokmanya Tilak Medical College and General Hospital
Mumbai, Maharashtra, India

Co-Editors

Dinesh Wade

MBBS MS (Obs/Gynae) DNB MRCOG (UK) FNB (Reproductive Medicine)
IVF Consultant
Department of Reproductive Medicine
Progenesis Fertility Center
Pune, Maharashtra, India

Manan Boob

MBBS MS (Obs/Gynae) DNB Fellowship in Advanced Gynaec Endoscopy
Consultant
Department of Obstetrics and Gynaecology
Shubham Hi-Tech Hospital
Amravati, Maharashtra, India

JAYPEE

JAYPEE BROTHERS MEDICAL PUBLISHERS

The Health Sciences Publisher

New Delhi | London

JAYPEE Jaypee Brothers Medical Publishers (P) Ltd

Headquarters
Jaypee Brothers Medical Publishers (P) Ltd
EMCA House, 23/23-B
Ansari Road, Daryaganj
New Delhi 110 002, India
Landline: +91-11-23272143, +91-11-23272703
+91-11-23282021, +91-11-23245672
Email: jaypee@jaypeebrothers.com

Corporate Office
Jaypee Brothers Medical Publishers (P) Ltd
4838/24, Ansari Road, Daryaganj
New Delhi 110 002, India
Phone: +91-11-43574357
Fax: +91-11-43574314
Email: jaypee@jaypeebrothers.com

Overseas Office
JP Medical Ltd.
83, Victoria Street, London
SW1H 0HW (UK)
Phone: +44 20 3170 8910
Fax: +44 (0)20 3008 6180
Email: info@jpmedpub.com

Website: www.jaypeebrothers.com
Website: www.jaypeedigital.com

Inquiries for bulk sales may be solicited at: jaypee@jaypeebrothers.com

Obs and Gynae PG Focus Series: Liver Disorders in Pregnancy

First Edition: **2025**

ISBN: 978-93-6616-271-3

Printed in India

Preface

The liver plays a crucial role in maintaining metabolic, haematologic, and immunologic homeostasis, functions that become even more significant during pregnancy. Pregnancy introduces unique physiological changes that can alter the presentation, progression, and outcomes of liver diseases. *Liver Disorders in Pregnancy* encompass a broad-spectrum—from relatively benign conditions such as intrahepatic cholestasis to potentially life-threatening complications like acute fatty liver of pregnancy or HELLP syndrome. Timely diagnosis and effective management of these conditions are essential to ensure the well-being of both mother and fetus.

This book, *Liver Disorders in Pregnancy,* is a comprehensive resource that addresses the complexities of liver disease in pregnancy. It covers pregnancy-specific liver conditions, the management of chronic liver diseases during pregnancy, and incidental findings that may arise in this period. Authored by experts in the field, the chapters provide up-to-date, evidence-based insights with a focus on clinical relevance and practical applications, making it an indispensable guide for those involved in the care of pregnant women.

A thorough understanding of liver disorders during pregnancy is critical for clinicians. These conditions often demand a multidisciplinary approach, requiring collaboration between obstetricians, hepatologists, and other specialists. This book aims to equip healthcare providers with the knowledge and tools needed to navigate these challenges effectively, ultimately improving maternal and neonatal outcomes.

We trust that this volume will serve as a valuable reference for understanding this intricate and essential subject, fostering better clinical decision-making and care strategies.

Editors
Komal N Chavan
Niranjan Chavan

Co-Editors
Dinesh Wade
Manan Boob

Acknowledgments

We express our gratitude to all those who contributed to the completion of this book on *Liver Disorders in Pregnancy*. This endeavor would not have been possible without the constant support of many individuals.

We are thankful to all the authors and co-authors for sharing their expertise and commitment to producing a resource of the highest standards.

We are grateful to our mentors and colleagues, whose valuable guidance helped us form the structure and contents of this book.

Our deepest gratitude to our families and friends for their unwavering support, patience, and encouragement during the demanding phases of this project have been our greatest strength.

We acknowledge the support of Shri Jitendar P Vij (Group Chairman) and Mr Ankit Vij (Managing Director) of M/s Jaypee Brothers Medical Publishers (P) Ltd, New Delhi, India, in publishing the book and their associates, particularly Ms Chetna Malhotra (Senior Director—Professional Publishing, Marketing, and Business Development), Ms Kritika Dua (Senior Commissioning Editor), and Ms Pragati Singh (Development Editor), who have been prompt, efficient, and most helpful.

Lastly, we hope that the postgraduate students find this book useful in their examinations and teachers for a quick revision. We also hope this book serves as a valuable resource, contributing to the betterment of patient care and surgical practice to the practicing obstetricians and gynaecologists.

Thank you all for being a part of this journey.

Contents

1 CHAPTER Anatomy of Liver

INTRODUCTION

Medical practitioners in antiquity have identified the liver as one of the three principal organs of the body, along with the heart and the brain. The Roman anatomist Galen identified the liver as the principal organ of the body arguing that it emerged first of all the organs in the formation of the fetus.

The liver is the largest organ in the body.

Its surface relations can be marked out by joining points on:

- The right costal margin in the midaxillary line (the 10th rib)
- The right 5th intercostal space
- The left 5th intercostal space in the midclavicular line.

In a healthy human being, the liver is not palpable. A palpable liver is suggestive of underlying pathology. On percussion, the dull node is felt over the hepatic surface.

By percussion, the mean liver size is 7 cm for women and 10.5 cm for men. A liver span 2–3 cm larger or smaller than these values is considered abnormal. The liver weighs 1,200–1,400 g in adult women and 1,400–1,500 g in adult men. It comprises 2.5% of the total body weight. The liver lies mainly in the right upper quadrant of the abdomen under the cover of 7–11 ribs on the right side occupying predominantly the right hypochondrium and the epigastrium.

SUPPORTS OF THE LIVER

- *Primary:* Inferior vena cava (IVC), hepatic veins, coronary ligaments, and triangular ligaments
- *Secondary:* Right kidney, right colonic angle, and duodenopancreatic complex
- *Tertiary:* Attachments of the liver to the anterior abdominal wall and diaphragm by the falciform ligament

ANATOMICAL FEATURES

The liver is divided into two surfaces—diaphragmatic/anterosuperior and visceral/posteroinferior. The liver is further divided into two major lobes—the right and the left lobe and two accessory lobes—caudate and the quadrate lobe. The liver has a border inferiorly.

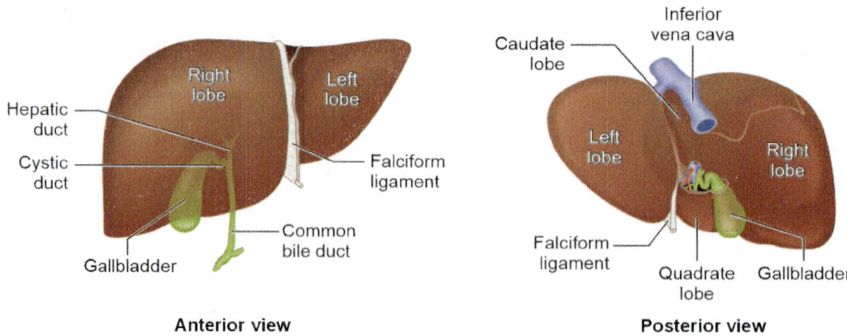

Fig. 1: Anatomy of liver: Anterior and posterior view.

The liver has two surfaces—the convex diaphragmatic surface and a relatively flat or even concave visceral or posteroinferior surface. The diaphragmatic surface of the liver is dome-shaped, smooth in the outline where it lies under the concavity of the inferior surface of the diaphragm. It separates from the pleura, pericardium, and lungs. The diaphragmatic surface of the liver is divided into the phrenic and the hepatorenal recesses. Subphrenic recess separates the diaphragmatic surface of the liver from the diaphragm. The right and left areas are divided by the falciform ligament which is derived from the ventral mesentery as shown in **Figure 1**. Hepatorenal recess is a part of the peritoneal cavity on the right side between the liver and the right kidney and the right suprarenal gland. The bare area of the liver is devoid of the peritoneum and directly in contact with the under-surface of the diaphragm.

LIGAMENTS OF THE LIVER

Falciform Ligament

A sickle-shaped fold of the peritoneum connects the anterior abdominal wall with the liver. The anterior border is attached to the under-surface of the diaphragm and the anterior abdominal wall. The posterior border is attached to the superior and the anterior surfaces of the liver. The free margin connects the umbilicus to the liver and it contains the round ligament of the liver or the ligamentum teres.

Anterior and Posterior Coronary Ligament

These attach the liver to the diaphragm. Two peritoneal ligaments are parts of the coronary ligament. The left triangular ligament is between the left lobe of the liver and the diaphragm. The right triangular ligament is between the right lobe of the liver and the diaphragm.

Round Ligament

Ligamentum venosum: Lesser omentum has two parts—hepatogastric ligament and hepatoduodenal ligament. Lesser omentum encloses the portal triad—bile duct, hepatic artery, and the portal vein. It passes from the liver to the lesser curvature to the stomach and 2 cm of the duodenum. The hepatogastric ligament extends from the porta hepatis to the lesser curvature of the stomach. Hepatoduodenal ligament extends from porta hepatis to the superior part of the duodenum and contains common bile duct, proper hepatic artery, and hepatic portal vein.

The visceral surface of the liver is covered with the visceral peritoneum except in the fossa of the gallbladder and the porta hepatis. The structures related to the visceral surface of the liver include the right anterior part of the stomach, the superior part of the duodenum, the lesser omentum, the gallbladder, the right colic, the right transverse colon, the right kidney, and the right suprarenal gland. Porta hepatis serves as the point of entry into the liver for the hepatic arteries and the portal vein and the exit point of the hepatic ducts.

LOBES

The major lobes of the liver are the right and the left lobe. The right lobe is the largest in volume and contributes to all the surfaces of the liver. In the diaphragmatic surface, it is divided from the left lobe by the falciform ligament superiorly and ligamentum venosum inferiorly. On the visceral surface, left sagittal fissure separates the two. The triangular smaller lobe that lies lateral to the left sagittal fissures and occupies the epigastrium and extends till the left hypochondrium is called the left lobe of the liver. Accessory lobes of the liver arise from the right lobe of the liver. The quadrate lobe is visible on the upper part of the visceral surface of the liver. Bounded on the left by fissure for ligamentum teres and on the right by the fossa for the gallbladder. Functionally related to the left lobe of the liver. The caudate lobe is visible on the lower part of the visceral surface of the liver and is bounded on the left by the ligamentum venosum and on the right by the groove for the IVC. Functionally, it separates from the right and the left lobes of the liver.

RELATIONS OF THE LIVER

- *Anteriorly:* Diaphragm, right and left costal margin, right and left pleura and lower margins of both lungs, xiphoid process and the anterior abdominal wall in the subcostal angle
- *Posterior:* Diaphragm, right kidney, hepatic flexure of the colon, duodenum, gallbladder, IVC, esophagus, and fundus of the stomach

Cantlie's Line

It grossly divides the liver into the left and right lobes using a plane from the gallbladder fossa to IVC. The major hepatic vein lies in the Cantlie's line. Couninaud divided the liver into functional right and left lobe by the main portal fissure containing the middle hepatic vein.

Portal Blood Flow

The liver has a dual blood supply. The hepatic portal vein brings 75–80% blood to the liver. The portal vein contains 40% more oxygen than the blood returning to the heart from the systemic circuit. The hepatic portal vein originates and ends in capillaries/venous sinusoids. It drains the abdominal part of the alimentary canal except for the lower part of the anal canal, spleen, and pancreas. It is devoid of valves and acts as a blood reservoir as shown in **Figure 2**.

Hepatic Veins

They form the basis for the lobar and the segmental anatomy. Hepatic veins drain peripherally and form the interlobar and intersegmental areas. Portal veins feed centrally and form the intralobar and intrasegmental areas. Major hepatic vein divides the liver into the right and the left lobe. The right hepatic vein divides the right lobe into the anterior and posterior segments. The left hepatic vein divides the left lobe into the medial and the lateral segment.

Nerve Supply

Parasympathetic supply is by the preganglionic fibers of the vagus nerve. Sympathetic innervations are by the postganglionic fibers from the celiac plexus.

Lymphatic Drainage

Lymphatics from the upper surface drain into the nodes in the posterior mediastinum. Lymphatics from the lower surface drain into hepatic nodes and the celiac nodes.

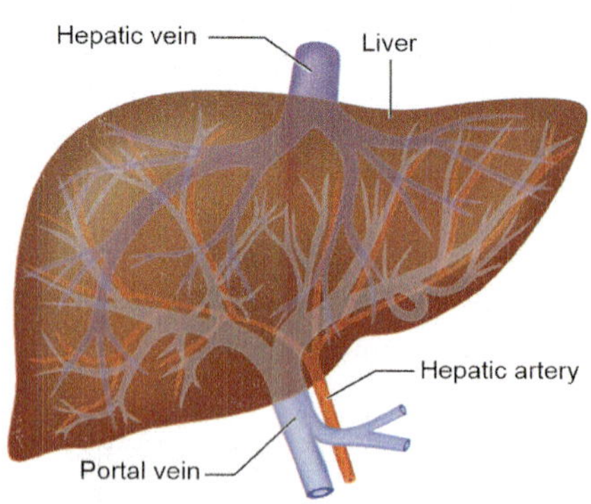

Fig. 2: Arteries and veins of liver.
Source: Kapoor VK. (2017). Liver Anatomy. [online] Available from: https://emedicine.medscape.com/article/1900159-overview. [Last accessed November, 2024]

CHAPTER 2

Physiology of Liver and Changes in Pregnancy

Changes in the value of certain serum liver function tests occur during normal pregnancy and an understanding of these physiological changes is necessary for the management of liver diseases. Because of the phenomenon of hemodilution, the albumin level decreases as early as the first trimester. Serum alanine and aspartate aminotransferase activity levels remain within the normal limits established for nonpregnant women. Measurement of serum aminotransferase levels thus remains the most useful test for the routine diagnosis of liver diseases during pregnancy. Serum total and free bilirubin concentrations are lower in pregnant women than in nonpregnant controls during all three trimesters, as are concentrations of conjugated bilirubin during the second and third trimesters. Serum alkaline phosphatase activity increases in late pregnancy, due both to the production of the placental isoenzyme and to the increase in bone isoenzyme. Consequently, measurement of serum alkaline phosphatase levels is not a suitable test for the diagnosis of cholestasis during pregnancy. Serum gamma-glutamyl transferase activity levels decrease during the second and third trimesters, and serum 5'-nucleotidase activity increases slightly in the second and third trimesters. Serum total bile acid concentrations during pregnancy are not different compared to levels in nonpregnant women. Measurement of serum bile acids may be useful for the diagnosis of cholestasis, especially when serum aminotransferase levels are within normal limits. In summary, according to the clinical setting, an increase in values of serum aminotransferase activity, serum GGT activity, serum bilirubin or fasting total bile acid concentrations during pregnancy should be considered pathologic.

INTRODUCTION

The pregnant woman experiences physiological changes to support fetal growth and development. The levels of estrogens (estradiol) and progesterone increase progressively during pregnancy. These sex hormones have effects on hepatic metabolic, synthesis, and excretory functions. The biliary excretion of bromosulfophthalein decreases during late pregnancy and the clearance of some compounds that are secreted into bile may therefore be impaired. The phenomenon of hemodilution secondary to the increase in plasma volume decreases the serum protein concentrations. Consequently, certain changes in values of liver function tests occur during normal pregnancy.

In this chapter, we review the liver-related clinical and biochemical changes that occur during normal pregnancy, with emphasis on liver function tests that are used for the management of liver diseases in pregnancy.

LIVER-RELATED SYMPTOMS AND PHYSICAL EXAMINATION IN PREGNANCY

Nausea and vomiting are common symptoms of early pregnancy and occur in over half of all pregnant women. The symptoms frequently persist throughout the day, although this condition was traditionally named "morning sickness". By contrast, *Hyperemesis gravidarum*, usually defined by severe vomiting beginning in early pregnancy and requiring hospitalization, is much less frequent. As discussed in Chapter 3, *Hyperemesis gravidarum* may be associated with liver involvement. Nausea or vomiting occurring during the second or third trimester should be considered pathologic and should require investigations including the measurement of serum aminotransferase activity. It should be noted that jaundice and generalized pruritus should never be considered normal features in pregnancy. Vascular spiders and palmar erythema are commonly associated with chronic liver disease and pregnancy.

In the United States of America, vascular spiders were found in 14% of white women by the 2nd month of pregnancy and in 66% by the 9th month of pregnancy. The frequency of these vascular spiders was noted to be lower in black women with 8% occurring in the 4th month of pregnancy and 14% in the 9th month. In this study, about three-quarters of the women had lost these vascular spiders by the 7th week after delivery. In the same study, palmar erythema was observed in 63% of the white women and 35% of black women. By the time of the postpartum consultation, palmar erythema had faded in all but 9% of the women. During pregnancy, these cutaneous vascular changes are not usually associated with hepatic dysfunction but may be related to sex steroids circulating in the blood over a long period. Physical examination of the liver is normal although it is difficult in late pregnancy because of the expanding uterus. In the postpartum period, after normal delivery, the liver and spleen may be palpable because of ptosis of these organs.

HEPATOBILIARY ULTRASONOGRAPHY IN PREGNANCY

Ultrasonography of the liver and biliary tract is widely used in the management of liver diseases outside pregnancy and is safe during pregnancy. In normal pregnancy, ultrasonographic examination reveals no dilatation of the biliary tract, but fasting gallbladder volume and residual volume after contraction are increased. The lithogenic or cholesterol saturation index of bile increases during pregnancy, which is considered a cholelithogenic state. Indeed, biliary sludge frequently occurs during pregnancy but is generally asymptomatic and often disappears spontaneously after delivery.

Gallstones are much less frequent (2% in an Italian study, 12% in a Chilean study) and may be associated with biliary pain. In the absence of suggestive symptoms, systematic ultrasound examination of the gallbladder as an extension of the routine pelvic ultrasound is not justified because silent stones in pregnant women need no treatment.

BLOOD VOLUME AND HEMODYNAMICS IN PREGNANCY

Plasma volume increases steadily from 6th to 36th week of gestation by about 50%. The red cell volume also increases, but the increase is moderate (about 20%) and delayed. Consequently, the total blood volume increases with hemodilution. The hematocrit decreases by the 24th week and becomes stable. Plasma and red cell volume decrease rapidly after delivery. This phenomenon of hemodilution should be kept in mind during the interpretation of all serum concentrations during pregnancy.

Cardiac output increases (about 40%) until the second trimester, then decreases and normalizes near term. Absolute hepatic blood flow remains unchanged, but the percentage of cardiac output to the liver decreases.

SERUM PROTEIN AND LIPID LEVELS IN NORMAL PREGNANCY

Serum albumin levels decrease during the first trimester, and this decrease becomes more accentuated as the pregnancy advances. The decrease in serum concentration is explained by the hemodilution phenomenon. Indeed, the intravascular mass of albumin is normal in pregnancy and the rates of synthesis or catabolism are unaltered in normal pregnancy compared to controls. By contrast, there is an increase in serum concentration of some proteins such as alpha-2-macroglobulin, alpha-1-antitrypsin, and ceruloplasmin. Fibrinogen and most coagulation factors (II, VIII, IX, and XII) increase when protein S levels decrease and fibrinolysis is inhibited. These physiological changes in hemostasis limit bleeding during delivery but are associated with an increased risk of thromboembolism during pregnancy and the postpartum period. Any change in the prothrombin time, which is widely used in the routine evaluation of chronic and acute liver failure, should be considered pathologic.

Serum cholesterol, triglyceride, and phospholipid concentrations increase in late pregnancy. This hyperlipidemia is a result of the metabolic adaptation to the pregnant state, saving glucose for the fetus. Except when a pregnant woman is suffering from acute pancreatitis, measurement of serum lipid concentrations is rarely useful during pregnancy. Serum concentrations of total globulins are unaffected by pregnancy.

SERUM LIVER FUNCTION TESTS IN NORMAL PREGNANCY

As outside pregnancy, serum liver function tests are essential in the management of liver diseases during pregnancy. Routine liver function tests usually include total and conjugated bilirubin, aminotransferases, alkaline phosphatase, and prothrombin time. In addition, gamma-glutamyl transferase (GGT) or 5'-nucleotidase may be used to confirm the hepatobiliary origin of increased levels of alkaline phosphatase. Measurement of serum bile acid concentrations may be useful for the management of cholestasis, especially during pregnancy. However, this test is not easily available and this limits its utilization. Awareness of the physiological changes in liver function tests is indispensable for the interpretation of these test values during pregnancy.

BILIRUBIN CONCENTRATIONS

Total bilirubin concentrations are decreased during all three trimesters of pregnancy. Free bilirubin concentrations have also been found to be lower in pregnant women than in nonpregnant controls during all three trimesters, as are concentrations of conjugated bilirubin during the second and third trimesters. Hemodilution could at least be partly responsible for the decrease in bilirubin concentration because albumin is the protein that transports bilirubin.

AMINOTRANSFERASE ACTIVITY

Measurement of serum alanine aminotransferase (ALT) and aspartate aminotransferase (AST) activity levels is the most useful test for the routine diagnosis of liver diseases. The effects of pregnancy in serum ALT and AST activity levels are somewhat controversial. In a few studies, a slight increase in ALT and/or AST activity has been found during the third trimester. However, in the majority of published studies, serum ALT and AST activity levels do not change during pregnancy or remain within the normal limits established in nonpregnant women. In one study, we found a slight increase in ALT during the second trimester of pregnancy compared to nonpregnant women, but all the values remained below the upper normal limit. We did not have any explanation for this slight increase in ALT and only during the second trimester in pregnant women compared to nonpregnant controls. An increase in ALT or AST levels during labor might be due to contractions of the uterine muscle. Thus, it should be emphasized that serum AST or ALT activity values above the upper normal limit before labor should be considered pathologic and should lead to further investigations.

ALKALINE PHOSPHATASE ACTIVITY

Serum alkaline phosphatase activity levels increase in late pregnancy, mainly during the third trimester. By contrast, serum alkaline phosphatase levels are lower in oral contraceptive users. This increase during pregnancy is not due to an increase in the hepatic isoenzyme but rather largely due to the production of the placental isoenzyme. During the third trimester, there is also an increase in the production of the bone isoenzyme as documented by an increase in its serum level up to 6 weeks post-delivery. These findings document that the measurement of serum alkaline phosphatase activity is not a suitable test for the diagnosis of cholestasis during late pregnancy and postpartum.

GAMMA-GLUTAMYL TRANSFERASE ACTIVITY

Serum GGT activity has usually been considered to be normal during pregnancy. When we compared serum GGT activity levels between pregnant women and nonpregnant women not taking oral contraception, we did not find a difference in the first trimester. However, we found a slight but significant decrease in GGT activity levels in the second and third trimesters in pregnant women. A significant decrease in serum GGT activity was also found in late pregnancy compared with early pregnancy in women with morning sickness. On the other hand, women suffering from viral hepatitis in early pregnancy have higher levels of serum GGT activity compared to women with viral hepatitis in late pregnancy, and the same has been observed in women taking oral contraceptives. These findings suggest that sex hormones may inhibit the hepatic synthesis of GGT, leading to a decrease in serum GGT activity in late pregnancy.

5′-NUCLEOTIDASE ACTIVITY

In two studies without control groups, no change was found in serum 5′-nucleotidase activity. In one study, serum 5′-nucleotidase activity was slightly higher in the second and third trimesters, compared with controls. A slight increase during the third trimester was also observed in two other studies. This slight physiological increase in serum 5′-nucleotidase during late pregnancy is a limitation for its use in the diagnosis of cholestasis.

BILE ACID CONCENTRATIONS

Increases in serum concentrations of certain bile acids have been reported during pregnancy, and it has been suggested that pregnancy could be associated with subclinical cholestasis. These changes in serum bile acids were minimal and observed mainly in the postprandial state. Moreover, some of these studies did not include a control group. By contrast, in a prospective study, fasting total bile acid concentrations measured during each trimester of pregnancy did not significantly differ from the control group. In clinical practice, when a woman experiences pruritus during pregnancy, the measurement of serum bile acid concentration may be useful for the diagnosis of cholestasis, especially when routine liver function tests are still within normal limits.

HISTOLOGICAL STUDIES

Standard and ultrastructural examination of the liver during normal pregnancy reveals no or minimal nonspecific abnormalities.

During normal pregnancy, except for alkaline phosphatase and 5′-nucleotidase, most values of serum routine liver function tests remain below the upper normal limits established in nonpregnant women. Thus, when liver disease is clinically suspected in a pregnant woman, any increase in serum ALT and AST activity levels, serum GGT activity, serum bilirubin, or fasting total bile acid concentrations should be considered pathologic and should prompt further evaluation.

3 CHAPTER Liver Function Tests

INTRODUCTION

The diagnosis of liver diseases depends on the combination of patient history, physical examination, laboratory testing, biopsy, and imaging studies such as ultrasound scan/computed tomography (CT)/magnetic resonance imaging (MRI) scans.

The liver function tests are used to detect:

- The presence of the liver disease
- Distinguish between different types of liver disorders
- Identify the extent of a known liver damage
- Follow the response to the treatment.

The following factors are to be noted before performing the liver function tests. The liver performs many biochemical and metabolic functions most of which cannot be quantified by any particular test. Enzymes are not very accurate in detecting liver function, moreover, they detect damage or interference with the blood flow. Interference must be performed within the context of the patients' risk factors, symptoms, concomitant conditions, medications, and physical findings. When one test provides abnormal findings or is persistently abnormal on serial determination—the probability of liver disease is high. When all the results are normal, the probability of missing occult liver disease is low.

Sample collection for liver function tests: Serum or plasma is to be collected. Avoid hemolytic or lipemic samples. Ensure adequate sample storage and transport. Samples to be collected in the plain red bulb. Safe biomedical practices to be followed.

CATEGORIZATION OF LIVER FUNCTION TESTS

- Tests based on detoxification and excretory functions
- Tests based on enzymes that reflect damage to hepatocytes
- Tests for enzymes that reflect cholestasis
- Tests that measure synthetic function

Tests based on detoxification and excretory functions:

- *Van den Bergh assay:* Determination of total, conjugated (direct), and unconjugated (indirect) bilirubin. Normal value of total <1–1.5 mg/dL. Normal value of direct bilirubin: up to 15% of the total (upper limit = 0.3 mg/dL). Total bilirubin activity decreases with gestational age.

Unconjugated bilirubin (UCB) levels are also lower in expectant mothers than in nonpregnant women in all three trimesters. In the first trimester, conjugated bilirubin (CB) levels are same in both the pregnant and nonpregnant women but the levels decrease in the second and the third trimester. Hemodilution in pregnancy explains partly the lower bilirubin concentration with advanced gestational age.

- *Isolated elevation of unconjugated bilirubin:* If the UCB is elevated, CB is <15%, watch out for hemolysis, if hemolysis is present then hemolytic disorders are suspected. If the hemolysis is absent with isolated elevation, the diagnosis is most likely Gilbert disease. Conjugated hyperbilirubinemia—liver or biliary tract disease. In most liver diseases, both the fractions are elevated.
- *Urine bilirubin:* Any bilirubin found in the urine is the conjugated bilirubin. Bilirubinuria implies the presence of liver disease.
- *Blood ammonia*: It is used for detecting hepatic encephalopathy and for monitoring hepatic synthetic function.

Tests for enzymes that reflect hepatocyte damage: Aspartate transaminase (AST) and alanine aminotransferase (ALT) remain within the normal range throughout the pregnancy. Uterine muscle contractions during labor may increase AST and ALT. Thus, serum AST and ALT values above the normal ranges in labor are therefore pathological need to be investigated further.

Aspartate transferase (AST/SGOT): Synthesized by the liver, cardiac muscle, skeletal muscle, kidneys, brain, pancreas, lungs, leukocytes, and red blood cell (RBC). Relatively nonspecific for liver damage.

Alanine transaminase (ALT/SGPT): Levels are increased in liver cell damage due to increased cell membrane permeability.

The rise in levels up to 300 U/L is nonspecific for any type of liver disorder. Levels >1,000 U/L are suggestive of extensive hepatocellular injury secondary to viral hepatitis, ischemic liver disease, drug- or toxin-induced damage. In most acute hepatocellular damage ALT >AST. AST:ALT >2:1 I and >3:1 are highly suggestive of alcoholic liver disease. Aminotransferase is not greatly elevated in obstructive jaundice.

Test for enzymes that reflect cholestasis:
Alkaline phosphatase (ALKP), 5'-nucleotidase (5'-NT), gamma-glutamyl transpeptidase (GGT): GGT has a more diffuse location and is less specific than ALP and 5'-NT.

Alkaline phosphatase—is a collection of isoenzymes present throughout the body. The clinically relevant forms are found in the liver, the biliary duct, white blood cell (WBC), small bowel, and placenta. Serum ALP is usually elevated in the third trimester and is mainly attributed to the placental isoenzyme than the elevation of the hepatic isoenzyme. Additionally, there is increased production of the bone isoenzyme with gestational age as a result of fetal bone development. It is elevated even in nonpathological causes. Alkaline phosphatase is not useful in distinguishing intra- and extrahepatic obstruction. Less than threefold increase is not specific for cholestasis (can be seen in almost any type of liver disorder). More than fourfold increase is significant and is associated with cholestatic liver disorder, infiltrative liver disease, and bone conditions associated with rapid bone turnover.

Tests that measure the biosynthetic function of the liver:
Serum albumin: It is synthesized exclusively by the hepatocytes. The half-life is 15–20 days. It is not a good indicator of acute/mild hepatic dysfunction. Serum albumin concentration decreases as the gestational age advances. Levels are affected minimally in viral hepatitis, drug-induced hepatitis, and obstructive jaundice. In hepatitis infection, if the albumin levels are <3 g/dL, they are suggestive of chronic liver disease. Other causes of hypoalbuminemia are protein malnutrition, protein-losing enteropathies, nephritic syndrome, and chronic infections.

Coagulation factors: All the clotting factors are exclusively synthesized in the liver except for factor VIII. Clotting factors have a rapid turnover rate. The half-life of factor VII is 6 hours and fibrinogen is 5 days which is shorter than albumin. Thus, the measurement of clotting factors is the single best acute measure of hepatic synthetic function.

Prothrombin time: It collectively measures II/V/VII/X. Biosynthesis of factors II/VII/IX/X depends on vitamin K. Prothrombin time (PT) may be elevated in hepatitis, cirrhosis, and disorders that result in vitamin K deficiency. Markedly elevated PT >5 seconds above the control not corrected by vitamin K is a poor prognostic sign in acute viral hepatitis and other acute and chronic liver diseases.

Normal values of liver function tests:

- *Bilirubin total:* 0–1 mg/dL
- *Conjugated bilirubin:* 0–0.35 mg/dL
- *Unconjugated bilirubin:* 0.2–0.65 mg/dL
- *SGOT:* 10–40 IU/L
- *SGPT:* 10–40 IU/L
- *Alkaline phosphatase:* 30–125 U/L
- *Total protein:* 6–8.5 g/dL
- *Serum albumin:* 3.5–5 g/dL
- *Serum globulin:* 2–3.5 g/dL
- *Gamma-glutamyl transpeptidase:*
    - 0–70 IU/L (male)
    - 0–40 IU/L (female)
- *Prothrombin time:* 10–13 seconds
- *International normalized ratio (INR):* 0.8–1.2

It is of utmost importance to consider normal reference ranges specific to pregnancy when interpreting LFT results which can be altered by the normal changes of pregnancy. Serum ALP and albumin decrease while ALT increases significantly with gestational age. Meanwhile, AST, GGT, and bilirubin fluctuate but remain within the normal ranges established in nonpregnant women. Hence, the normal gestation-related alterations, patients history, and presenting complaints are to be taken into account before interpreting the LFT. Changes in liver function tests in different liver disorders are shown in **Table 1**. **Flowchart 1** shows the diagnostic pathway for liver disease.

TABLE 1: Changes in liver function tests in different liver disorders in pregnancy.

	Acute hepatitis	*ICP*	*HELLP*	*AFLP*
Serum ALT and AST	Moderately high	Normal to mild rise	Moderately high	Moderately high
Serum alkaline phosphatase	Normal to mild rise	High	Normal	Normal
Platelets	Normal	Normal	Low	Normal

(AFLP: acute fatty liver of pregnancy; ALT: alanine aminotransferase; AST: aspartate transaminase; HELLP: hemolysis and elevated liver enzymes and low platelets; ICP: intrahepatic cholestasis of pregnancy)

Flowchart 1: Diagnostic pathway for liver disease.

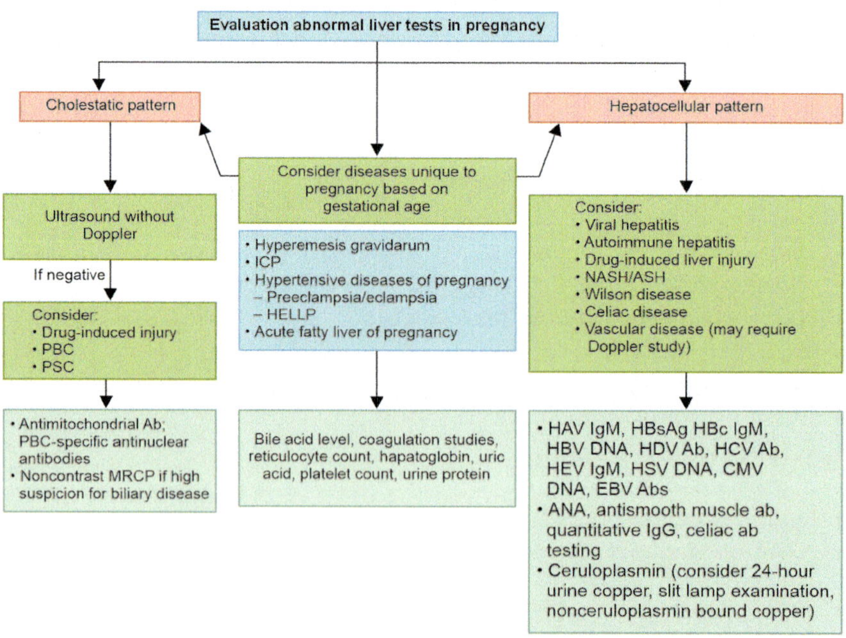

(HELLP: hemolysis and elevated liver enzymes and low platelets; ICP: intrahepatic cholestasis of pregnancy)

4

CHAPTER

Intrahepatic Cholestasis of Pregnancy

INTRODUCTION

Intrahepatic cholestasis of pregnancy (ICP) is one of the rarest obstetric multifactorial disorders that occurs most commonly during the third trimester of pregnancy and can lead to adverse maternal and fetal outcomes. It is also known as obstetric cholestasis, recurrent jaundice of pregnancy, pruritus gravidarum, icterus gravidarum, and idiopathic jaundice of pregnancy. It was first described by Ahlfeld in 1883 as a pregnancy-induced disorder that presents with maternal pruritus, jaundice, raised hepatic transferases, and bile acid levels in the last trimester reverting to normal within 2–3 weeks postdelivery.

EPIDEMIOLOGY

Owing to the recent medical advances, the incidence of ICP has considerably reduced among all the ethnic groups to <2% of all the live births. The reported incidence of ICP in Asia, North America, and Australia is <1%, while it is 1.2–1.5% in Indian Asian and Pakistani–Asian origin. Several decades ago, ICP was more common among the Araucanos Indians of Chile (27.6%) and Aymara Indians of Bolivia (13.8%). It is commonly seen to be associated with twins and multiple pregnancies with a recurrence risk of 25% in the subsequent pregnancy.

ETIOLOGY AND PATHOGENESIS

The etiology of ICP is still investigational and not completely understood. The implication of genetic, hormonal, and environmental factors has been proposed in the etiopathogenesis of ICP. ABCB4 (MDR3) is a crucial hepatocellular phospholipid transporter that facilitates the secretion of the major human phospholipid, phosphatidylcholine into bile. 15% of cases of ICP are attributed to the mutations in this transporter. Other nonsignificant bile salt export pumps ABCB11, aminophospholipid transporter F1C1, and ATP8B1 are less commonly associated with the pathogenesis of ICP. Genetic predisposition of ICP is supported by familial clustering, geographical and ethnic variation, and a high rate of recurrence in subsequent pregnancies. The hormonal influence of estrogens, progesterone, and their metabolites has been strongly associated with the development of ICP.

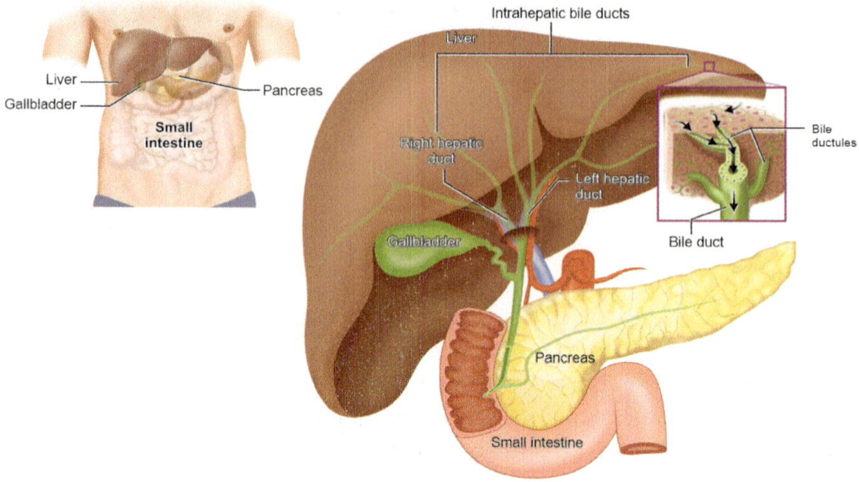

Fig. 1: Anatomy of intrahepatic bile ducts.
Source: MedlinePlus. Intrahepatic cholestasis of pregnancy. [online] Available from https://medlineplus.gov/genetics/condition/intrahepatic-cholestasis-of-pregnancy/. [Last accessed November, 2024]

Development of ICP is seen more commonly in the last trimester, when the endogenous production of estrogen is high. An association of ICP with multiple pregnancies and a history of high dose of exogenous estrogen use as a contraceptive among women with a personal or family history of ICP suggest the estrogenic influence for the development of ICP. In in vitro studies, it was found that estrogens impaired the basolateral and canalicular bile acid transporter expression of liver cells by transcriptional mechanisms as shown in **Figure 1**. Patients with ICP have significantly raised levels of progesterone, mono- and disulfated progesterone metabolites, and an increased ratio of 3-alpha-hydroxylated steroids to 3-beta-hydroxylated steroids. Exogenous factors like nutritional deficiency and selenium deficiency have been associated with the development of ICP.

CLINICAL MANIFESTATIONS

The clinical importance of obstetric cholestasis lies in the potential fetal risks which include spontaneous or iatrogenic preterm birth and intrauterine fetal demise. Pruritus is seen in 23% of pregnancies of which only a very small proportion will be having ICP.

Pruritus is the main clinical symptom of ICP which can be mild or severely disabling thereby affecting the patients quality of life by causing chronic fatigue, sleep deprivation, and suicidal thoughts. Pruritus worsens in the evening without the development of any specific skin lesions with a predominance for the palms and the soles. The lesions are shown in

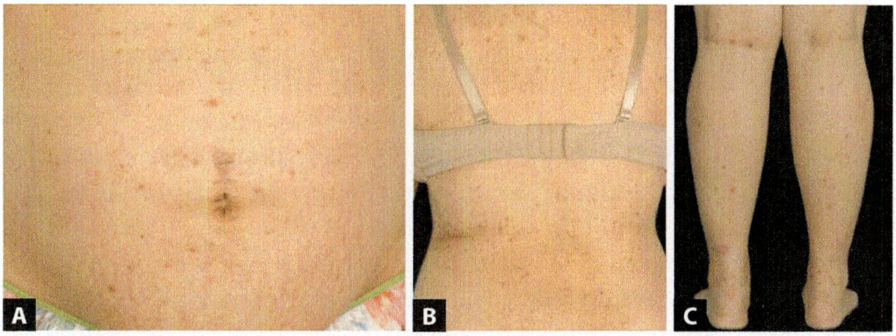

Erythematous papules and nodules on the abdomen (A), back (B), and legs (C)

Figs. 2A to C: Dermatological lesions in intrahepatic cholestasis of pregnancy.
Source: Oh CC, Oon H. (2018). Intrahepatic cholestasis of pregnancy. [online] Available from https://www.mdedge.com/dermatology/article/176979/mixed-topics/intrahepatic-cholestasis-pregnancy. [Last accessed November, 2024]

Figures 2A to C. Trauma due to intense scratching (dermatographia artefacta) which is seen in ICP should be differentiated from other common skin conditions like eczema or atopic eruption of pregnancy. Pemphigoid gestationis and pleomorphic eruption of pregnancy should be considered if the rash is present. It usually presents after 30 weeks of gestation but can present as early as 6 weeks in certain atypical cases. Very rarely jaundice is the initial presenting symptom, it usually develops 4 weeks after the pruritus sets in with moderate elevation of hepatic aminotransferases and conjugated bilirubin. Abdominal pain, malaise, and vomiting are the other vague presenting symptoms. Patients with ICP are more commonly associated with gallstone formation and cholecystitis. Pale stools, dark-colored urine, jaundice, and other risk factors for the development of ICP like family history of ICP, multiple pregnancies, presence of gallstones, and carriage of hepatitis C virus should be identified.

DIAGNOSTIC INVESTIGATIONS/BIOCHEMICAL MARKERS

Pregnancy-specific ranges for the liver function tests should be used. For transaminases, gamma-glutamyl transferase, and bilirubin, the upper limit of normal throughout the pregnancy is 20.5 which is lower than the nonpregnant range. In patients with persistent unexplained pruritus and normal liver function, liver function tests should be repeated every 1–2 weeks. The normal level of bile salts does not exclude the diagnosis of ICP.

Liver function tests and maternal fasting bile acid levels are the keys to the diagnosis of ICP. Serum total bile acid levels may increase 10–100 times above the normal value. Maternal fasting bile acid levels of >40 micromole/L have been associated with high fetal complications. In ICP, the ratio of serum cholic acid to chenodeoxycholic acid increases whereas the ratio of glycine to taurine conjugated bile acid falls. In ICP, the serum bile acid composition of women displayed a more hydrophobic pattern with higher levels of lithocholic acid and unconjugated serum bile acids. In 20–60% of patients presenting with pruritus, hepatic transferases are elevated to 2–10-fold. In 50% of patients, serum glutamyl transpeptidase is normal or modestly elevated up to four times the normal upper limit. Typically, the hepatic transferases will range from just above the upper limit of normal to several hundred. Once the diagnosis of ICP is established, LFTs should be monitored weekly until delivery. In a normal pregnancy, LFTs may increase in the first 10 days of the puerperium, hence in the case of ICP postnatally the LFT measurement should be deferred till at least 10 days and done at the time of the next follow-up visit. Postnatal resolution of symptoms and biochemical abnormalities are mandatory for the diagnosis of ICP. Serum alkaline phosphatase though elevated up to 7–10 times are difficult to interpret due to the placental isoenzyme. To summarize, the diagnosis of ICP is based on the following four features—(1) pruritus, (2) absence of other diseases that cause pruritus or jaundice, (3) elevated fasting serum bile acids of >10 micromole/L, and (4) spontaneous relief of signs and symptoms within 2–3 weeks after the delivery. Liver biopsy is nonspecific and nondiagnostic. Histopathology in ICP reveals noninflammatory centrilobular cholestasis, bile plugs in hepatocytes, and canaliculi without bile duct dilatation and injury. To exclude the other causes of deranged liver function tests, viral screen for hepatitis of A, B, C, Epstein–Barr virus and cytomegalovirus, liver autoimmune screen for chronic active hepatitis, antismooth muscle, and antimitochondrial antibodies for primary biliary cirrhosis and liver ultrasound should be done.

DIFFERENTIAL DIAGNOSIS

Due to the nonspecific clinical presentation and biochemical markers, many other disorders may be misdiagnosed as ICP during pregnancy, hence a high index of suspicion is warranted to make a correct diagnosis. The differential diagnosis of ICP with pruritus and elevated serum bile acids include skin diseases, dermatoses of pregnancy, renal pruritus, allergic reactions, polycythemia rubra vera, and malignancies like Hodgkin's lymphoma. Hyperemesis gravidarum should be the first differential diagnosis of ICP with elevated liver enzymes in the first trimester. HELLP (hemolysis and elevated liver enzymes and low platelets) syndrome, preeclampsia, eclampsia, and acute fatty liver of pregnancy are the closest differentials of ICP in the third trimester presenting with elevated hepatic enzymes. In all the trimesters, ICP should be differentiated from all forms of viral hepatitis, alcoholic, drug-induced hepatitis, biliary obstruction, primary sclerosing cholangitis, and primary biliary cirrhosis.

MANAGEMENT

Alleviating maternal symptoms and improving fetal outcomes is the primary objective of pharmacological treatment in the ICP. Blunt topical emollients like calamine lotion and aqueous menthol are safe in pregnancy and can provide relief from pruritus. Systemic treatments aimed at relieving pruritus like cholestyramine, chlorpheniramine, activated charcoal, and guar gum are not recommended due to insufficient evidence. The efficacy of S-adenosyl methionine for the control of maternal symptoms and improving fetal outcomes is not established and hence not recommended for the treatment of ICP. Currently, the hydrophilic bile acid, ursodeoxycholic acid (UDCA), is the most effective treatment for the ICP. Several randomized controlled trials have established the supremacy of ursodeoxycholic acid over cholestyramine and dexamethasone in the treatment of cholestasis of pregnancy. UDCA therapy is more commonly associated with effective reduction in pruritus, lowering of hepatic transferases and bile acid levels and term delivery. UDCA is better tolerated by pregnant women and no adverse effects in the mothers and the newborns have been seen. The exact mechanism of UDCA in relieving the symptoms and reducing the impact of ICP has not been completely understood. UDCA improves hepatocellular secretion by posttranscriptional stimulation of canalicular expression of the key transport proteins. UDCA restores the impaired maternal placental bile acid transport across the trophoblast. As vitamin K is fat-soluble, malabsorption secondary to biliary obstruction or hepatic disease can lead to vitamin K deficiency, which is required for the production of coagulation factors 2, 7, 9, and 10. Water-soluble vitamin K is widely used in the management of ICP. Women should be counseled about the need for water-soluble vitamin K (menadiol sodium phosphate in the dose of 5–10 mg daily), if the prothrombin time is prolonged. Postnatal vitamin K should be offered to the babies in a usual way.

The current additional risk of stillbirth in ICP above that of the general population is not determined but is likely to be small. Women with ICP should be counseled about the increased incidence of meconium (30–44%), premature delivery (7–25%), fetal distress, need for operative intervention in the form of caesarean section (10–36%), and postpartum hemorrhage (2–22%). The risk of intrapartum meconium passage is inversely proportional to the period of gestation and directly proportional to the serum levels of bile acids. It was concluded that the risk of meconium passage increases linearly with a 19.7% increase for every 10 micromoles/L increase in total bile acid concentration. Current clinical evidence is inconclusive in strongly establishing the association between the raised hepatic enzymes, bile acids with adverse fetal outcomes, although high bile acid levels are related to the passage of meconium, sudden intrauterine fetal demise, prematurity, abnormal cardiotocograph, and fetal asphyxia events. Thereby it was concluded that poor fetal outcomes cannot be entirely predicted by the biochemical results and hence the delivery decisions should be individualized. Ultrasound and antenatal fetal monitoring are not reliable methods for predicting fetal compromise in obstetric cholestasis, hence the pregnancy with obstetric cholestasis should be regarded as a high-risk pregnancy and continuous intrapartum fetal monitoring should be offered to all the patients. Fetal death in ICP is usually sudden and nonpredictable as placental insufficiency, fetal growth restriction, oligohydramnios, and umbilical artery Doppler abnormalities are not the features of the disease.

Induction of labor in the 37th–38th week of gestation has been recommended to reduce the risk of perinatal mortality as conventional antepartum testing does not reliably predict fetal mortality. The timing and risks of delivery should, therefore, be individualized with the involvement of a well-trained obstetrician and neonatologist. The implications of obstetric cholestasis should be clearly understood. The patient should be reassured about the lack of long-term maternal or fetal sequelae, high risk of recurrence 45–90% in the next pregnancy, contraceptive choices usually avoiding the estrogen-containing methods and the increased risk of ICP among the other family members. LFTs to be done 6 weeks postdelivery and a detailed hepatic evaluation 8 weeks postdelivery is proposed. The RCOG and the British Liver Trust have patient information leaflets of obstetric cholestasis. There is also an Obstetric Cholestasis support group (*http://www.ocsupport.org.uk/*).

5

CHAPTER

Acute Fatty Liver of Pregnancy

INTRODUCTION

Acute fatty liver of pregnancy (AFLP) was first described by Sheehan in 1940 as acute yellow atrophy of the liver. It is a rare but potentially hazardous disorder that occurs in the third trimester or the early postpartum period. The incidence of this complication is 1 in 10,000–15,000 pregnancies. With prompt diagnosis and treatment, maternal and perinatal mortality has been decreased from 75% and 85% to 18% and 23%, respectively.

ETIOLOGY

The currently available data does not conclusively establish the cause of this disorder but mitochondrial dysfunction is the most likely studied cause of AFLP. Beta-oxidation of the fatty acids occurs in the mitochondria which requires four enzymatic reactions. The special carrier transport proteins transport the fatty acids from the outer to the inner mitochondrial membrane where they are broken down by the enzymes to generate energy. The pathway is utilized to generate energy in the vital organs when the glycogen stores are depleted. Hence, the deficiency of the third enzyme long-chain 3-hydroxyacyl-CoA dehydrogenase (LCHAD) results in the accumulation of the medium and long-chain fatty acids. The first association between LCHAD deficiency and recurrent AFLP was proposed by Schoeman et al. in 1991. LCHAD deficiency is inherited in the autosomal recessive manner. The most common recognized mutation occurs in the alpha unit of the trifunctional protein gene in which the glutamic acid at the 474 positions is replaced by glutamine and this is associated with 65–90% of the LCHAD deficient patients. As the mutation is recessive, when both the parents are heterozygous for this mutation and the fetus acquires both these mutations, the fetus will be unable to oxidize long-chain fatty acids. These unmetabolized free fatty acids return via the placenta to the maternal circulation which puts an additional strain on the maternal hepatic enzyme activity thereby causing AFLP. The toxic products of the LCHAD deficiency accumulate in the mitochondria and cause fatty infiltration and degeneration of the muscle fibers and this affects both cardiac and skeletal muscle development. LCHAD deficiency usually presents clinically in the neonatal period or early childhood mostly after a period of fasting or prolonged illness associated with hyperbilirubinemia. Infants can present with liver failure,

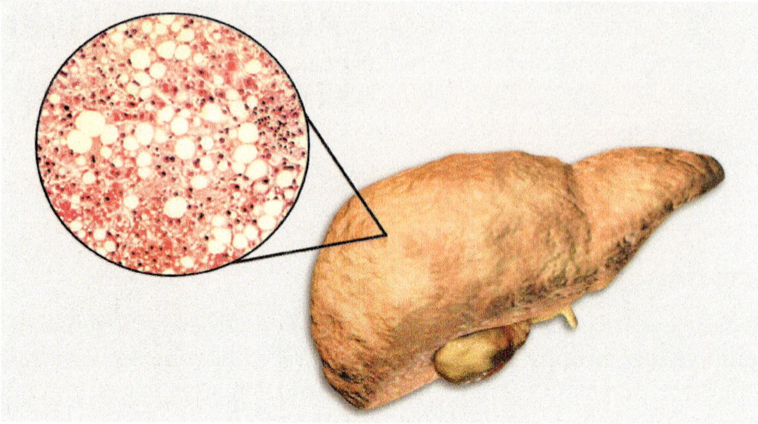

Fig. 1: Gross and microscopic image of fatty liver in pregnancy.
Source: https://www.istockphoto.com/photo/fatty-liver-liver-steatosis-gm858263750-141648693

severe cardiomyopathy, hypoketotic hypoglycemic encephalopathy, and pigmentation of the fundus of the eye which may be nonreversible.

PATHOPHYSIOLOGY

Due to impaired beta-oxidation of the fatty acids, there is microvesicular fatty infiltration of the hepatocytes. The fat content of the liver may increase from the normal 5 to 13–19% in AFLP. Accumulation of toxic metabolites along with ammonia production and fatty accumulation eventually causes coagulopathy and hypoglycemia evolving into hepatic failure. Due to hepatocytolysis and atrophy of the liver cells, the liver is small, soft, and yellow as shown in **Figure 1**.

RISK FACTORS

Though LCHAD deficiency is a major causative factor for the development of the AFLP and other factors also predispose to the development of AFLP. Ethnicity and dietary factors have no role in the development of AFLP. Primigravid status, preeclampsia, male fetus, and multiple gestations are some of the high-risk factors. In a heterozygous mother (for LCHAD mutation) carrying a homozygous fetus, the nonsteroidal anti-inflammatory drug containing the salicylates inhibits the trifunctional protein and the long-chain fatty acid oxidation in the mitochondria which may precipitate the development of AFLP.

CLINICAL PRESENTATION

The AFLP usually presents in the third trimester with the mean gestational age being 35–36 weeks, some cases can present as early as 22 weeks of gestation.

As there is a wide spectrum of symptoms of AFLP, the clinical diagnosis may be difficult. Patients present with nonspecific symptoms such as anorexia, malaise, nausea, vomiting, abdominal pain, and headache. The patient may be febrile and present with jaundice in the majority of the cases. The liver is usually tender, small, and nonpalpable. The common signs and symptoms of the acute fatty liver of the pregnancy are jaundice (70%), abdominal pain radiating to the right hypochondrium, epigastrium and the back (50–60%) altered sensorium and disorientation (60–80%), disseminated intravascular coagulation (55%), nausea and vomiting (50–60%), gastrointestinal bleeding (20–60%), and acute renal failure (50%). AFLP can have a disastrous effect on the fetus. Maternal metabolic acidosis secondary to the impaired clearance of lactate by the damaged hepatocytes directly affects the fetal acid–base status and is essential for fetal well-being.

LABORATORY DIAGNOSIS

The Swansea criteria is used for diagnosing AFLP. According to this criteria, six or more of the following findings are required in the absence of another cause:

1. Vomiting
2. Abdominal pain
3. Polydipsia/polyuria
4. Encephalopathy
5. Elevated bilirubin >14 μmol/L
6. Hypoglycemia <4 μmol/L
7. Elevated urea >340 μmol/L
8. Leukocytosis >11 × 10/L
9. Ascites or bright liver on ultrasound scan
10. Elevated transaminases [aspartate aminotransferase or alanine aminotransferase (AST or ALT)] >42 IU/L
11. Elevated ammonia >47 μmol/L
12. *Renal impairment*: Creatinine >150 μmol/L
13. *Coagulopathy*: Prothrombin time >14 seconds or activated partial thromboplastin time (aPTT) >34 seconds
14. Microvesicular steatosis on liver biopsy.

Diagnosis of AFLP may be challenging as the patient's history, clinical features, and biochemical abnormalities may mimic other conditions such as acute viral hepatitis, preeclampsia, HELLP (hemolysis, elevated liver enzymes, low platelet count) syndrome, intrahepatic cholestasis. As AFLP is uncommon in pregnancy, pregnant women with liver dysfunction first rule out all the common causes. While AFLP can be confused with preeclampsia due to the overlapping features, hypoglycemia and jaundice are not seen in preeclampsia. AFLP usually presents acutely with severe coagulopathy which is not seen in preeclampsia. Viral hepatitis is associated with positive serological markers and elevated transaminases well above 1000 u/L which is not seen in AFLP. Intrahepatic cholestasis of pregnancy is associated with intense pruritus, raised bile acids, and elevated alkaline phosphatase and is not associated with vomiting, abdominal pain, nausea, or vomiting. A liver biopsy should not be done to confirm the diagnosis of AFLP due to the risk of complications arising due to underlying coagulopathy. Microvesicular fatty infiltration of the liver can be identified by using special stains such as Oil Red O. Histologically, there is microvesicular steatosis with sparing of zone 1 with patchy hepatocellular necrosis as shown in **Figure 1**.

MANAGEMENT

Due to the diagnostic dilemma associated with AFLP, a high level of suspicion with a low threshold for admission is required. Early diagnosis, immediate delivery, and intensive supportive care are the foundations in the treatment of AFLP. Patients with additional obstetric and medical high-risk factors leading to multiorgan dysfunction and death should be admitted immediately without any delay for extensive maternal and fetal monitoring. Maternal stabilization that includes airway management, correction of electrolytes, underlying coagulopathy, underlying hypoglycemia, hypertension treatment, adequate administration of blood and blood products, and maternal vital sign assessment, should be ensured. A multidisciplinary approach involving the critical care specialist, gastroenterologist, and perinatologist is preferred. Once the maternal stabilization is achieved, expedite the fetal delivery. A vaginal approach is preferred but a caesarean section can be considered for obstetric indications and because of rapidly deteriorating maternal and fetal status. In the postpartum period, intense hemodynamic monitoring is required due to underlying coagulopathy, hypoglycemia, and electrolyte imbalance. The other potential complications of AFLP which usually occur after the onset of hepatic and renal dysfunction, e.g., pancreatitis should be anticipated and not ignored. Serial measurement of serum lipase and amylase several days after onset of hepatic dysfunction may help in avoiding these complications. Pseudocysts and hemorrhagic pancreatitis may be diagnosed using magnetic resonance imaging/computed tomography (MRI/CT) scan. Liver transplantation is rarely required in AFLP except in certain grave cases presenting with irreversible fulminant hepatic failure, hepatic encephalopathy, severe metabolic acidosis, or liver rupture complicated by hepatic necrosis where orthoptic liver transplantation may be the only life-saving measure. The risk of recurrence of AFLP is 25–35% in the subsequent pregnancy, hence the women planning to conceive again should be counseled for early antenatal registration with a skilled obstetrician and intensive care unit (ICU) facilities.

CHAPTER 6

Viral Hepatitis in Pregnancy

INTRODUCTION

The most common cause of jaundice in pregnancy is acute viral hepatitis. Hepatitis can be caused by diseases exclusively associated with pregnancy as well as those not exclusively associated with pregnancy. Diseases uniquely associated with pregnancy include hyperemesis gravida, acute fatty liver of pregnancy, severe preeclampsia and HELLP (hemolysis, elevated liver enzymes, and low platelet count) syndrome, and intrahepatic cholestasis of pregnancy.

Hepatitis A

Hepatitis A is a positive sense, single-stranded RNA (ss RNA) virus. It belongs to the family Picornaviridae. Transmission of this virus is by the fecal-oral route. Infection is more prevalent in developing countries with poor sanitation leading to water and food contamination. The average incubation period of the hepatitis A virus (HAV) is 30 days. It is seen in the highest concentration in the feces, serum, and saliva in descending order. The infection can also be transmitted through sexual contact through any oral interaction. Intrauterine, bloodborne, and perinatal transmission of hepatitis A is rarely seen. It causes acute infection without any chronic sequelae.

Epidemiology

It is very prevalent in developing countries with an incidence of 1:1,000. The disease is self-limited. Mortality is low 0.3–0.6%.

Hepatitis B

It is an enveloped double-stranded DNA virus as shown in **Figure 1**. It has circular DNA, belongs to the family Hepadnavirus, and is mainly transmitted through the blood-borne route and contaminated body fluids. It does not cross the placenta thereby fetal infection occurs only when there are breaks in the maternal-fetal barrier. 50% of cases worldwide are attributed to perinatal transmission. In pregnant women with chronic hepatitis B infection and positive hepatitis B e-antigen (HBeAg), there is a 90% chance of newborns being infected with the hepatitis B virus (HBV). HBeAg is suggestive of higher infectivity and virulence. High titers of HBV

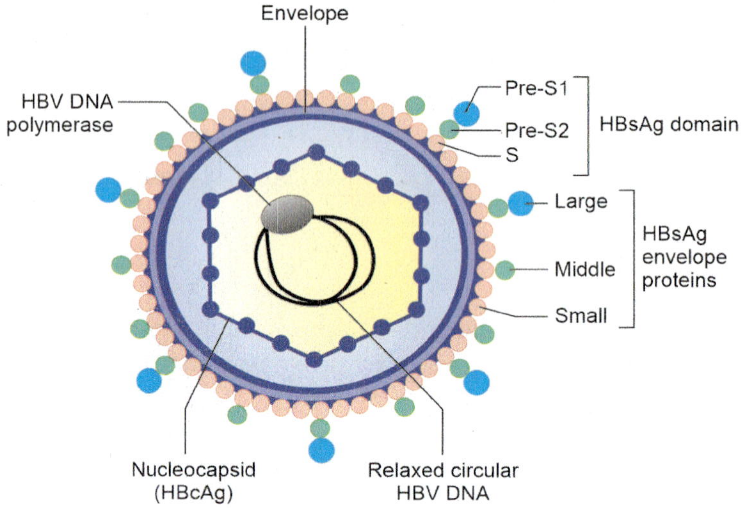

Fig. 1: Structure of hepatitis B virus.

DNA are suggestive of higher viral load. Chronic HBV infection is associated with cirrhosis and hepatocellular carcinoma.

Epidemiology

It is the most common cause of chronic hepatitis worldwide. 65 million women of childbearing age are infected with chronic HBV. The prevalence of chronic HBV among pregnant women in the United States is 0.7–0.9%.

Hepatitis C

Hepatitis C virus (HCV) is a partially double-stranded, plus-sense RNA virus. It has 11 major genotypes and 15 different subtypes. Acute infection occurs during the first 6 months after exposure. Failure to clear the HCV beyond 6 months would lead to the development of cirrhosis and hepatocellular carcinoma. Vertical transmission is the major mode of maternal to child transmission. Perinatal transmission of HCV occurs in the last month of pregnancy or delivery. Other modes of transmission include infected blood products, transfusion of contaminated blood and blood products, intravenous drug users, sharing needles, and sexual contact. Fetoinvasive procedures such as amniocentesis, chorionic villous sampling, and cordocentesis which are likely to break the maternal-fetal barrier increase the risk of transmission of hepatitis C during pregnancy and delivery.

Epidemiology

About 8% of pregnant women are affected by HCV. The prevalence of HCV infection in the united states among antenatal mothers is 1–2.5%.

Hepatitis D

It is caused by the hepatitis delta virus (HDV). It has a single-stranded circular RNA. It is a defective virus with an incomplete RNA that requires the assistance of HBV specifically hepatitis B surface antigen (HbsAg) for being infectious. The major mode of transmission is by the parenteral route whereas vertical transmission is rare. Coinfection of HDV and HBV leads to severe acute infection. Superinfection of HDV on a chronic HBV leads to higher progression to chronic hepatitis D infection.

Epidemiology

The prevalence of HDV is 20% in pregnant women with chronic HBV infection.

Hepatitis E

Hepatitis E virus (HEV) is an icosahedral, nonenveloped. It has a single-stranded positive RNA. It belongs to the family Hepeviridae. There are seven types of HEV of which one to four infect humans. The main mode of transmission by fecal-oral route is seen in developing countries with poor sanitation. Vertical transmission of HEV is seen between 23 and 50%. Genotype 3 causes sporadic cases, especially in an immunocompromised state. It is rarely transmitted through sexual intercourse.

Epidemiology

Hepatitis E viral infection is responsible for 7,000 deaths and 3,000 still-births. It mainly affects the women in the second and the third trimesters. As there is a very high risk of progression to fulminant hepatitis with hepatitis E infection, the mortality rate with this infection in pregnancy ranges from 5 to 25%.

SYMPTOMATOLOGY

Acute viral hepatitis in pregnancy can present with variable symptoms or in asymptomatic in the majority of the cases. Most of the symptoms caused by the various viral hepatitides are variable and overlapping. Symptoms may be as nonspecific as fever, abdominal pain, nausea, vomiting, diarrhea, malaise, and dark colored urine. In women with hepatitis B and C infection in which the risk of chronicity is the highest, patients may present with critical symptoms such as decompensated cirrhosis, coagulopathy, esophageal variceal bleeding, and hepatic encephalopathy.

LABORATORY DIAGNOSIS

The liver function tests are the most common first-line investigations that are performed when the patient presents with hepatitis. During the acute episodes of infection, alanine transaminase (ALT), aspartate transaminase

(AST), and alkaline phosphatase are elevated 2–100 folds. International normalized ratio (INR), prothrombin time (PT), and serum ammonia levels are evaluated for the diagnosis of acute and chronic viral hepatitis.

Hepatitis A

Hepatitis A viral infection is diagnosed by the detection of the presence of anti-HAV immunoglobulin M (IgM) in the pregnant women and the newborn as IgM is suggestive of acute infection. Screening should be done for all pregnant women who have been in contact with persons infected with acute hepatitis A infection.

Effects of Hepatitis A Infection in Pregnancy

The HAV infection is seen uncommonly during pregnancy and is not associated with serious adverse outcomes. However, serious cases of HAV may be associated with preterm labor, placental abruption and premature rupture of the membranes. When HAV infection is associated with fever and hypoalbuminemia, an aggressive clinical course is expected. HAV is not usually associated with maternal mortality or perinatal transmission. Infants born to mothers with HAV infection have normal antibody and transaminase levels. In extremely rare cases where maternal to child transmission of HAV infection occurs, there is a risk of fetal ascites, meconium peritonitis, and distal ileum perforation.

Breastfeeding in Hepatitis A Infection

Breastfeeding should be encouraged in mothers who are infected with HAV infection. The infant should be protected through the administration of immunoglobulin or inactivated vaccine. Even though the mothers infected with HAV infection have anti-HAV antibodies and HAV RNA in the breast milk, the evidence does not support the transmission of HAV to infants through suckling.

Prevention of Hepatitis A Infection

Hygienic practices such as handwashing with safe water, avoiding contaminated food and drinking water, and avoiding unpeeled fruits and vegetables are the only effective measures for controlling the transmission of HAV infection. If, unimmunized pregnant women are visiting HAV endemic or underdeveloped countries, they need to be protected against hepatitis A infection. Hepatitis A vaccine is prepared from the inactivated virus and is considered safe in pregnancy. It is available in the monovalent form or as a combination with the HBV vaccine. There should be clear indications for administering the vaccine to pregnant women. As the incubation period of HAV infection is 15–50 days, the vaccine should be administered before travel to ensure adequate protection.

Hepatitis B

The US Preventive Services and the American Congress of Obstetricians and Gynecologists (ACOG) recommend universal screening for HBV infection at the first antenatal visit and at any time during pregnancy if any symptoms of hepatitis are seen.

Serology of hepatitis B infection as explained in **Table 1**.

- *Hepatitis B surface (HBs) antigen:* It is a protein on the surface of the HBV. It can be detected in high levels in serum during acute or chronic HBV infection. Its presence indicated that the affected individual is infectious. The human body produces antibodies to HBsAg as a part of a normal B cell-mediated humoral immune response. HbsAg is the antigen used to make the hepatitis B vaccine.
- *Hepatitis B surface antibody (anti-HBs):* Recovery from a recent infection and immunity is indicated by the presence anti-HBs. Anti-HBs antibody is also seen in subjects who have been completely immunized against hepatitis B infection.

TABLE 1: Interpretation of hepatitis B serological markers.

HBsAg Anti-HBc Anti-HBs	Negative Negative Negative	Susceptible
HBsAg Anti-HBc Anti-HBs	Negative Positive Positive	Immune due to natural infection
HBsAg Anti-HBc Anti-HBs	Negative Negative Positive	Immune due to hepatitis B vaccination
HBsAg Anti-HBc Ig M Anti-HBc Anti-HBs	Positive Positive Positive Positive	Acutely infected
HBsAg Anti-HBc Ig M Anti-HBc Anti-HBs	Positive Positive Negative Positive	Chronically infected
HBsAg Anti-HBc Anti-HBs	Negative Positive Negative	Unclear interpretation: • Resolved infection, most common • False positive anti-HBc, thus susceptible • Low level chronic infection • Resolving acute infection

(CDC)
(HBc: hepatitis B core antibody; HBs: hepatitis B surface antibody; HBsAg: hepatitis B surface antigen)

- *Total hepatitis B core antibody (anti-HBc):* Anti-HBc appears at the onset of the infection and persists for life. Its presence indicates previous ongoing infection with the HBV. The antibody for HBV core antigen remains positive throughout life.
- *IgM anti-HBc:* In cases where IgM anti-HBc is positive, it indicates recent and acute hepatitis B infection <6 months.

Effects of Hepatitis B Virus in Pregnancy

Hepatitis B virus infection is not known to cause increased teratogenic effects in pregnancy. However, the incidence of low birth weight and prematurity are higher in acute hepatitis B infection while the chronic HBV infection is associated with gestational diabetes mellitus, antepartum hemorrhage and prematurity. The acute infection needs to be differentiated from the other causes which include intrahepatic cholestasis of pregnancy, acute fatty liver of pregnancy, or preeclampsia. The main risk of chronic hepatitis B infection is the rupture of esophageal varices and subsequent bleeding (25%) that occurs in the second trimester. Other grave risk factors include hepatic decompensation, rupture of splenic aneurysm, and jaundice. In patients with chronic liver infection and cirrhosis, if the various are absent before pregnancy, all patients should undergo endoscopic screening for the presence of varices in the second trimester. If the varices are large enough, beta-blockers (propranolol) should be used despite the fetal effects. Acute variceal bleeding is managed by endoscopic intervention as in nonpregnant patients. Diuretics, rifaximin, lactulose, and hepatoprotective diet are given for the management of hepatic encephalopathy and ascites. In large parties, vaginal delivery is preferred over caesarean section due to the perioperative risk.

Effect of Pregnancy on Hepatitis B Virus Infection

Immunomodulatory changes in pregnancy are due to the effects of progesterone. There is a shift in the immunity toward TH2 from TH1 with an increased amount of regulatory T cells which lead to a suppressed immune response against HBV. These immune modifications mainly aim to prevent fetal rejection. Due to the above immune adaptations in pregnancy, there is increased viral HBV DNA expression and a reduction in the levels of aminotransferases.

Perinatal Hepatitis B Virus Transmission

Perinatal transmission of HBV is very commonly seen. When the baby has a hepatitis B infection due to perinatal transmission, the HBsAg is positive for 6 months after the birth. Anti-HBe antibody and Anti-HBc antigen which cross the placental barrier disappear at 12 and 24 months of age, respectively. Hence, their presence merely indicates a passive transplacental transfer

Flowchart 1: Algorithm for management of hepatitis B in pregnancy.

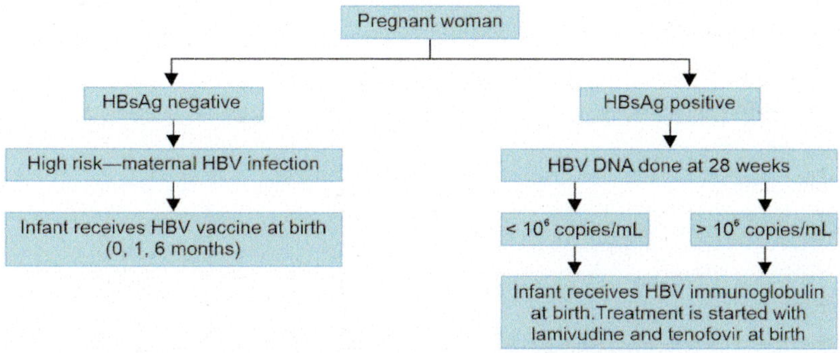

(HBsAg: hepatitis B surface antigen; HBV: hepatitis B virus)

and not HBV infection status. When the mother is immunized, the risk of perinatal transmission is very high and variable, it ranges from 70 to 90% for HBeAg positive mothers, 25% for HBeAg negative/HBeAb negative mothers, and 12% for HBeAg negative/anti-HBeAg positive mothers. All the women are screened antenatally at their first visit for HBsAg antibodies. If a mother is found to be HBsAg positive, the babies receive passive-active prophylaxis at birth to reduce vertical HBV transmission. Active prophylaxis involves the administration of the hepatitis B vaccine and passive immunoprophylaxis involves hepatitis B immunoglobulin administration. Despite taking adequate measures of passive-active immunoprophylaxis in women who are HBsAg positive, around 3–13% of the babies born to these mothers especially when the HBeAg is positive become chronic HbsAg carriers. The maternal HBeAg positive serological status and a high viral load have a positive correlation with the intrauterine transmission of HBV. Lower levels of HBeAg expression are associated with lower levels of viral replication and a lower risk of intrauterine HBV transmission. The algorithm for management of hepatitis B in pregnancy is shown in **Flowchart 1**.

Treatment of Hepatitis B Virus during Pregnancy

The decisions regarding the treatment of HBV infection in the pregnancy should include the consideration of the maternal and fetal high-risk factors. The possible risk of short and long-term liver disorder outcomes in the mother and the teratogenic effects of the various drugs on the fetus should be considered before starting the treatment. US Food and Drug Administration (US FDA) has approved seven drugs for the treatment of hepatitis B infection in pregnancy as given in **Table 2**.

The choice of anti-HBV drug to be given in pregnancy depends on the aim of the treatment whether it is to treat active liver disease for which therapy cannot be delayed or to prevent perinatal transmission of infection. In women who become pregnant while on anti-HBV therapy, whether the drug

TABLE 2: Drugs approved for the treatment of hepatitis B virus infection in pregnancy.

Drug	*Pregnancy category*
Lamivudine	C
Entecavir	C
Telbivudine	B
Adefovir	C
Tenofovir	B
Interferon alpha-2B	C
Pegylated—interferon alpha-2c	C

in use should be stopped, continued, or changed to another class B drug. When the woman is in the immunotolerant phase of the infection (high HBV DNA levels, normal transaminases and normal liver biopsy), the treatment can be started after the delivery without any hurry. However, in HBeAg positive women with high viral load, third-trimester prophylaxis could be initiated to reduce the perinatal transmission. In a pregnant woman who is already on anti-HBV treatment, if there is a risk of significant fibrosis, the therapy should be continued by choosing the least teratogenic agent to reduce the risk of decompensated liver disease.

Management of Hepatitis B Virus in Pregnancy

Every woman should be screened for hepatitis B infection in the first trimester. If she is negative and at low risk of infection, there is no need for routine vaccination. If she is negative and at a high risk of infection, she should be vaccinated. In a woman who is positive for hepatitis B infection, understanding the disease status is very important. If the HBsAg positive woman with active HBV infection (elevated ALT and a very high viral load) with suspected cirrhosis, therapy should be initiated irrespective of the trimester. If the woman has the inactive disease (low ALT and less viral load), therapy is not required but continuous surveillance is suggested because of the risk of the flare of hepatitis B in the later pregnancy and a few months of postpartum. Quantification of the viral load by HBV DNA testing should be done if all women tested positive for hepatitis B infection at 28 weeks. Depending on the number of HBV DNA copies, she should be offered anti-HBV treatment. There is no convincing evidence to suggest the advantage of elective caesarean section over normal vaginal delivery in hepatitis B positive mothers. The role of elective caesarean section in preventing maternal to child transmission of hepatitis B is not well established.

Breastfeeding in Pregnancy

Breastfeeding is not contraindicated in HBV-infected mothers who are not on antiviral therapy and if the infants receive immunoprophylaxis. For the mothers who are on antiviral therapy with lamivudine or tenofovir, breastfeeding is not advisable because of the little data available about the safety of antiviral exposure during breastfeeding.

Hepatitis C in Pregnancy

The HCV RNA is detected in saliva, urine, menstrual fluid, breast milk, and semen. There is no vaccine to prevent HCV infection, neither antiviral nor immunoglobulin is recommended. The overall risk of vertical transmission is 5.2% and the incidence is 0.33%. The risk of vertical transmission of HCV is enhanced by high levels of HCV RNA titers, concomitant human immunodeficiency virus (HIV) infection, and multiple risk factors.

There is no association between vertical transmission and gestational age, mode of delivery, chorioamnionitis, subsequent pregnancies, and breastfeeding. To prevent maternal-fetal transmission, obstetric preventive measures need to be employed if the maternal viral load is high and no adequate antiviral treatment has been initiated. Invasive fetal procedures such as chorionic villous sampling, fetal blood sampling, and placement of scalp electrodes should be avoided.

Most women infected with HCV are asymptomatic. There is no deleterious effect of pregnancy on the course of HCV infection. Hepatitis C infection in pregnancy is not associated with increased abortion rates, lower birth weights, stillbirths, or congenital malformation. The risk of prematurity is increased if the hepatitis is acquired in the last trimester. There is an increased risk of obstetric cholestasis in women infected with HCV.

Antenatal screening should be performed in all women at their first visit. Mothers with chronic HCV infection should be immunized against HAV and HBV as superinfection can have adverse consequences. Screening should be done by detection of HCV antibody. Persistent HCV antibody levels indicate persistent infection rather than immunity. Anti-HCV if positive then HCV RNA testing should be done. Women with HCV positive status should be counseled thoroughly about the associated maternal and fetal risks, risks of vertical transmission of infection, and infant protection strategies. Interferon plus ribavirin is the first-line treatment for HCV infection. Women who are exposed to interferon inadvertently should continue the pregnancy. In chronic hepatitis, interferon administration can be delayed. According to the American Society for Reproductive Medicine (ASRM) 2004 guidelines, interferon administration in pregnancy is not advisable. In acute hepatitis C infection, interferon should be considered with close monitoring. As ribavirin is FDA category

X drug, it should not be used in pregnant women, women attempting pregnancy or their male partners. The role of elective caesarean section in minimizing the risk of transmission is not established hence it is not recommended primarily for the prevention of the transmission. If vaginal delivery is attempted then frequent per vaginal examinations, early membrane rupture, fetal scalp electrodes, and fetal scalp blood sampling should be avoided. HCV RNA is found in a very tiny amount in breast milk and hence unable to infect newborns. Breastfeeding is not contraindicated in mothers with HCV infection. Most infants delivered to HCV-infected mothers (106 copies/mL) progress to hepatitis. All the children born to women who are infected with HCV should be screened for this virus. Transplacentally transferred HCV antibodies can persist in the infant for up to 15 months. polymerase chain reaction (PCR) testing of the infant at 3 months and 6–12 months provides the most conclusive evidence about the presence or absence of infection in the infant.

HEPATITIS E IN PREGNANCY

Hepatitis E is a waterborne pathogen transmitted by the fecal-oral route. HEV infection during pregnancy in the third trimester can result in fulminant hepatitis and causes increased maternal and fetal morbidity and mortality. The incubation period of the virus ranges from 5 to 64 days. The rate of vertical transmission of the HBV virus is 50%. Out of all the genotypes, type 1 is associated with severe infection, fulminant hepatic failure, and maternal death. Due to immunomodulation that occurs in pregnancy, there are suppressed immune responses during pregnancy. Infection with type 1 genotype is associated with 15–25% mortality. Hepatitis E infection in pregnancy is associated with higher rates of preterm delivery, preterm premature rupture of membrane (PPROM), operative intervention, and neonatal complications with prolonged maternal and fetal ICU stay. At present, although there is no consensus to treat patients with HEV infection in pregnancy early fetal delivery should be planned. The clinical presentation of HEV infection is variable and associated with jaundice, anorexia, tender hepatomegaly, abdominal pain and tenderness, nausea, vomiting, and fever. Cases of chronic HEV infection have been reported in immunosuppressed people. HEV reactivation can occur in immunocompromised individuals. Diagnosis of HEV infection is based on the detection of specific antibodies to the virus in the blood. RT-PCR and immune electron microscopy can be used to detect the HEV. There is no proven treatment for HEV infection. Prevention is the only effective approach against the disease. As hepatitis E is self-limiting, only symptomatic treatment is required. However, in pregnancy all the women may be offered admission to

TABLE 3: Differential diagnosis of liver disorders in pregnancy.

	Acute hepatitis	*ICP*	*HELLP*	*AFLP*
Trimester	Any trimester	Third	Third	Third
Presenting symptoms	Fever, jaundice	Pruritus	Hypertension, nausea, vomiting, and pain	Nausea, vomiting, and abdominal pain
Serum ALT and AST	Moderately high	Normal-to-mild rise	Moderately high	Moderately high
Serum alkaline phosphatase	Normal-to-mild rise	High	Normal	Normal
Platelets	Normal	Normal	Low	Normal
Fetal complications	Transmission of infection in HBV and HCV	Prematurity, fetal distress, and IUGR	IUGR, prematurity	Premature delivery

(AFLP: Acute fatty liver of pregnancy; ALT: alanine transaminase; AST: aspartate transaminase; HBV: hepatitis B virus; HCV: hepatitis C virus; HELLP: hemolysis, elevated liver enzymes, and low platelet count; ICP: intracranial pressure; IUGR: intrauterine growth restriction)

provide appropriate treatment, monitoring for maternal and fetal well-being, assessment of progression to fulminant hepatitis, and emergency intervention if the need arises **(Table 3)**.

7

CHAPTER

Chronic Liver Disorders in Pregnancy

INTRODUCTION

In women with cirrhosis and portal hypertension, with a compensated liver function, conception is a rare event. Maternal and fetal outcomes are better with extrahepatic portal venous obstruction (EHPVO) and noncirrhotic portal fibrosis as compared to cirrhosis of the liver with compensated liver function. Maternal mortality in patients with cirrhosis ranges from 2 to 18% whereas perinatal mortality is between 11 and 18% due to intrauterine growth restriction or IUGR. A nephrotic syndrome that occurs secondary to chronic liver disease in 0.025% of all pregnancies further results in uteroplacental insufficiency. With the rising incidence of cirrhosis and portal hypertension complicating the pregnancies, a holistic approach by an experienced obstetrician and a multidisciplinary approach is required.

MATERNAL AND FETAL RISKS

The incidence of cirrhosis in pregnancy is very rare, with 1 in 9,590 pregnancies. Cirrhosis of the liver results in many metabolic and hormonal imbalances that lead to anovulation and amenorrhea and makes conception difficult. Malnutrition and altered hepatic metabolism of sex steroids are contributory. Infertility usually reflects the degree of hepatic dysfunction and in well-compensated cases, fertility is preserved. As pregnancy is associated with altered hemodynamics like, increased cardiac output, decreased peripheral vascular resistance, there is worsening of portal hypertension and increased risk of variceal bleeding. This may be accompanied by severe anemia, hepatic encephalopathy and dysfunction, splenic aneurysm rupture, ascites, spontaneous bacterial peritonitis, and postpartum hemorrhage. The highest risk of active variceal bleeding is seen in the second and third trimester of pregnancy and in the second stage of labor where Valsalva's maneuver and bearing down is done aggravates the risk of variceal bleeding. Variceal bleeding is noted in 50% of cases of portal hypertension and 30% cases of cirrhosis in pregnancy. The maternal mortality rate with cirrhosis and decompensated liver function is as high as 18% whereas in noncirrhotic portal hypertension the rates are between 6 and 12%. The causes of death include hematemesis, postpartum hemorrhage, and hepatic coma. Perinatal outcomes are usually poor in women with liver disease such as IUGR, prematurity, stillbirth, anasarca, polyhydramnios, acute kidney injury, chronic renal failure, gestational hypertension, preeclampsia, and eclampsia.

MANAGEMENT

Antenatal

In well-compensated liver disease, pregnancy is not contraindicated. MELD (models for end-stage renal disease) is used for assessing the severity of liver disease. Patients with a MELD score of ≤6 should be counseled about the minimal significant complications and those with a MELD score of >10, should be advised against pregnancy. After the basic antenatal workup patients who have conceived should be counseled about the high-risk nature of the pregnancy. The case should be handled by an experienced obstetrician with the involvement of surgeons, gastrointestinal medicine, and critical care experts. Liver and renal infection tests, haematological assessment should be done weekly till the end of the second trimester and repeated twice weekly in the third trimester. Patients should be offered inpatient admission for appropriate fetal and maternal monitoring twice weekly from the second trimester onward. Empirically, anemia should be treated as it leads to cardiac compromise. The main aim is to prevent the poor pregnancy outcome that is associated with sudden and massive variceal bleeding, endoscopic ligation of the varices should be considered in the second trimester. Nonselective beta-adrenergic blockers like propranolol reduce the risk of variceal bleeding by 50% but may be associated with adverse fetal complications such as fetal bradycardia and fetal growth restriction. When the bleeding is too extensive to be controlled by endoscopic measures, an emergency transjugular portosystemic shunt may be done as a life-saving measure. In the presence of cirrhosis, existent portal hypertension, and nephritic syndrome, nonsteroid drugs like aspirin should be avoided as they may preprecipitate acute renal failure and decompensation. Pregnant women with cirrhosis are more vulnerable to the development of ascites and spontaneous bacterial peritonitis and hence should be treated with third-generation cephalosporins. In case of progressive liver failure or advanced decompensation, early pregnancy termination should be considered, otherwise, the pregnancy can be allowed to go to term in case of well-compensated liver disease. Antenatal steroids should be given for planned pregnancy termination before 34 weeks. The Asian Pacific Association for the Study of the Liver (APASL) recommends that women with EHPVO can be allowed vaginal delivery, caesarean section is only reserved for obstetric indications. As such, caesarean section over vaginal delivery to reduce the risk of variceal bleeding in the second stage of labor is not recommended currently by any studies.

Peripartum

Sufficient blood and blood products should be arranged for with the facilities for balloon tamponade. Labor can be induced and augmented normally using prostaglandin and oxytocin respectively. The second stage of labor should be shortened to prevent undue bearing down, thereby reducing the risk of variceal bleed. Epidural analgesia is preferred. The third stage of labor should be actively managed and methergine should be associated. Methergine is associated with a sudden rise in blood pressure and a high risk of variceal rupture. There is a higher risk for spontaneous abortion, premature birth, stillbirths, and perinatal death in women with portal hypertension.

Postpartum

Antibiotics should be judicially used and individualized keeping in mind the risk of hepatotoxicity and teratogenicity. Breastfeeding is not usually contraindicated. Contraception in the form of intrauterine devices, barrier methods should be advised. Permanent sterilization may not be advisable due to underlying coagulopathy. Hormonal contraception should be avoided as it may cause cholestasis.

Keeping in mind the maternal and fetal outcomes associated with chronic liver disease, a multidisciplinary approach in a tertiary care center with the availability of intensive care units should be considered for desirable outcomes.

8

CHAPTER

Liver Malignancy and Pregnancy

INTRODUCTION

Liver tumors can be classified into benign and malignant.

BENIGN TUMORS

The common benign tumors of the liver include hepatic hemangioma, hepatic adenoma, and focal nodular hyperplasia. Other rare benign tumors include fibroma, lipoma, leiomyoma, and cystadenoma.

Hepatic Hemangioma

A liver hemangioma is a tangle of blood vessels in or around the surface of the liver. It is the most common benign tumor in adults and children and is more frequently seen in the right lobe of the liver than the left lobe. They are noncancerous in nature. They are congenital is the origin and frequently diagnosed between 30 and 50 years. They are seen more frequently among women than men. Women on hormonal therapy with elevated estrogen levels are at a higher risk for developing hemangiomas than women who are not on hormonal medications. Most of the time, they are diagnosed incidentally but they can present with pain in the right upper quadrant of the abdomen, postprandial fullness, nausea, vomiting, and lack of appetite. Hemangiomas can be aggravated by an injury or fluctuating estrogen levels. Ultrasound, computed tomography (CT) scan or magnetic resonance imaging (MRI) can be used for diagnosing hemangiomas. Most hemangiomas do not require any treatment, however, if symptomatic surgical resection with hepatic artery embolization can be done.

Hepatic Adenoma

It is an unusual benign tumor with a high tendency of intraperitoneal rupture and bleeding inside the abdominal cavity. 90% of hepatic adenomas are seen in women in the age group of 20–40 years and are strongly associated with elevated estrogen levels secondary to hormonal contraceptives intake. When hepatic adenomas increase in size beyond 6–8 cm, they are considered cancerous and are at risk of developing into hepatocellular carcinoma. Usually, asymptomatic and nonpalpable. Less frequently they can present with right-sided hypochondriac pain (30%), palpable hepatomegaly, and risk of intraperitoneal bleeding (30%) which may be associated with hypotension, tachycardia, and sweating. It is important to distinguish hepatic adenomas from hemangiomas and focal nodular hyperplasia because of the higher risk of progression to malignancy in hepatic adenomas. MRI and a polyphasic CT scan can be used in differentiating them. Patients with adenomas should avoid estrogen-containing oral contraceptives and hormonal replacement therapy. Pregnancy is attributed to elevated estrogen levels which may cause the adenoma to grow faster, so patients with hepatic adenomas should avoid pregnancy.

Focal Nodular Hyperplasia

It is the second most common benign tumor of the liver which is a result of congenital arteriovenous malformation. There is an abnormal hepatocyte response where all the normal constituents of the liver are present but in an abnormal pattern despite which the liver can perform a normal function.

MALIGNANT TUMORS

The most frequent malignant primary liver cancer is a hepatocellular malignancy which in most cases are metastases from other tumors, especially the gastrointestinal tract. Other rare primary liver malignancies include cholangiocarcinoma, mixed tumors, sarcoma, and hepatoblastoma.

Risk Factors for Liver Malignancy

The most important risk factors vary from country to country. In countries where hepatitis B is endemic (China), hepatitis B is the predominant cause of the development of liver cancer. In Unites States due to higher vaccination rates, the risk of hepatitis B infection is low and hence the major cause of hepatocellular carcinoma (HCC) in hepatitis C and liver cirrhosis. Hepatitis B and C infections globally contribute to 25% of cases of hepatocellular carcinoma. The risk of HCC in type 2 diabetes is seven times higher than in nondiabetics depending on the duration of diabetes and the treatment protocol followed. Chronic alcoholism contributing to liver cirrhosis is a major risk factor in the development of hepatocellular carcinoma. Other risk factors include aflatoxins, nonalcoholic steatohepatitis, hemochromatosis, Wilsons disease, and autoimmune hepatitis.

Signs and Symptoms

Hepatocellular carcinoma can present with a wide range of symptoms. The nonspecific symptoms include right upper quadrant pain, nausea, vomiting, malaise, and palpable lump in the abdomen. Severe symptoms suggestive of the aggressive course include ascites, easy bruising due to underlying coagulopathy, ascites, loss of appetite, and unexpected weight loss.

Diagnosis

The diagnosis can be made by taking a detailed history, use of hepatotoxic drugs, viral markers, history of alcohol abuse, ultrasonography, and triple-phase CT scan. Alpha-fetoprotein and des-gamma-carboxyprothrombin levels can be measured to make the diagnosis.

Prognosis

The usual outcome is very poor as only 20% of the carcinomas can be completely removed using surgery. If the tumor is not resected completely, the disease recurrence with aggravation of the disease status is seen in the next 3–6 months. Survival is variable, and in cases where the complete resection is possible survival, is usually >6 months.

Prevention

Childhood vaccination against hepatitis B can prevent the development of hepatocellular carcinoma. Restricted alcohol intake, adequate control of diabetes, avoiding red meat in the diet, and hepatotoxic agents are the other preventive measures. Genetic screening for hemochromatosis is another adjunct in early risk assessment for the development of hepatocellular carcinoma.

LIVER MALIGNANCY AND PREGNANCY

Risk Factors and Etiopathogenesis

The incidence of HCC in pregnant women is 1 in 100,000 most of whom are of African or Asian origin. Among the Asian and the African race, hepatitis B virus and oral contraceptives were the main etiologies for the development of HCC during pregnancy. Pregnancy seems to accelerate the development of liver tumors. The fulminant course of HCC in pregnancy is attributed to two main etiologies—estrogen elevation which accelerates the evolution of HCC and pregnancy-induced immunosuppression. HCC in pregnancy is associated with fetal loss in 42% of cases. The risk of HCC increases with parity but the overall incidence of HCC is low among reproductive years and infertility secondary to cirrhosis. Early menarche, late menopause, multiparity, and oral contraceptive pills are risk factors for the development of HCC which again suggest a negative impact of pregnancy on HCC. Estrogen causes hepatocyte mitosis, hypervascularity, free radicals, which reactivate HBV and decrease humoral immunity. Family history of HCC is seen in only 8% of the cases.

Clinical Presentation and Laboratory Findings

The HCC is asymptomatic in the early stages of pregnancy. Right upper quadrant pain, palpable mass, weight loss, or hepatomegaly has been the most common presenting symptoms. Rare cases may also present with nausea, vomiting, and abnormal liver enzymes. Elevated alpha-fetoprotein levels in a pregnant patient with a normal fetus are indicative of maternal disease especially HCC, however, AFP screening is not very specific in diagnosing HCC as it depends on multiple variables such as maternal weight, age, diabetes, and ethnicity, though elevated AFP levels have a very high positive predictive value. Other laboratory abnormalities include hyperbilirubinemia, prolonged prothrombin time, hypoalbuminemia, and elevated hepatic transaminases.

Management

Liver resection is the only best possible management in liver malignancies presenting during pregnancy. In a woman presenting at early gestation, medical termination of pregnancy should be offered and beyond that delivery should be expedited to ensure early and prompt management of HCC. HCC during pregnancy has a poor outcome and nearly 20% of the cases present with distant metastasis at the time of presentation. The fibrolamellar variety of HCC has a better prognosis. If the normal pregnancy course is followed, delivery by caesarean section occurs in 44% of cases and live births are seen in only 58% of the cases.

Solid organ malignancies should not be missed in pregnancy and should be approached meticulously. The women with a family history of cancer presenting with unusual manifestations should be thoroughly scrutinized.

9

CHAPTER

Liver Transplantation in Pregnancy

Don't take your organs to heaven, heaven knows we need them here.

INTRODUCTION

Liver transplantation is the only life-saving option in patients with advanced liver disease. Acute irreversible fulminant hepatic failure secondary to preeclampsia, viral/autoimmune or drug-induced hepatitis, acute fatty liver of pregnancy, hepatic encephalopathy, and acute liver rupture are some of the cases where liver transplant might seem indispensable to the patient's life. Ever since the first pregnancy in a transplant recipient in 1958, pregnancy in the recipients of solid organ transplants is increasingly common. The first successful pregnancy in the liver graft recipient was reported in 1978. When the transplant is performed in the background of decompensated cirrhosis, pregnancy is unlikely due to infertility, anovulation, and secondary amenorrhea. Pregnancy in a postliver transplant failure should be regarded as a high-risk case and the counseling should include the optimal time for planning the pregnancy, appropriate contraception methods, management of immunosuppression in pregnancy, and the fetomaternal outcomes in women conceiving postliver transplantation.

PRECONCEPTION PLANNING

Chronic severe liver disease disturbs the hypothalamic-pituitary-ovarian axis causing hypogonadotropic hypogonadism leading to anovulation and secondary amenorrhea in 50% of the cases thereby preventing successful spontaneous conception in end-stage liver disease. The etiology of hypogonadism in chronic liver disease is multifactorial mostly attributed to the malnutrition that is seen in cirrhotic patients. The current literature suggests that though the menstrual function returns to normal within 3 months following the liver transplantation, conception should be delayed for 1 year for improved maternal and fetal outcomes. There is no recommendation by the American Society for Transplantation for a time interval between transplantation and conception, positive prognostic factors such as lack of rejection episodes in the previous year, adequate and stable graft rejection, and stable immunosuppressant dosing should be considered while counseling the patients who are anxious for conception.

CONTRACEPTION

Presently, there are less data regarding the safest and the most effective contraception following liver transplantation for the prevention of an unwanted pregnancy. Barrier methods have the lowest theoretical risk for systemic interactions and are much safer than other methods in postliver-transplant patients. Combined oral contraceptive pills are traditionally associated with mild hepatic dysfunction and gall stones and reversible cholestasis hence they are preferably not advised in postliver transplant recipients. While transdermal patches with minimum systemic effects can be used as contraception. Intrauterine devices are not the contraception of choice in liver transplant recipients mainly because the immunosuppressants used can interfere with the efficacy of the intrauterine device and increased the rate of pelvic infection.

IMMUNOSUPPRESSION IN PREGNANCY

Calcineurin inhibitors (cyclosporine and tacrolimus) suppress the T-cell function by inhibiting interleukin 2. They are classified as US Food and Drug Administration (US FDA) category C and are relatively safe to be used in pregnancy. The side effects include maternal diabetes, hypertension, preeclampsia, renal dysfunction, and perinatal hyperkalemia.

Azathioprine

Azathioprine is a purine antimetabolite resulting in the suppression of cell-mediated immunity. It is used extensively in inflammatory bowel disease and rheumatological disease. There are not many adverse fetal effects as the fetal liver lacks the enzymes inositol pyrophosphorylase which is required for the conversion of azathioprine metabolites 6-mercaptopurine into its active component thiouric acid. It is US FDA category D with no reported obvious teratogenic effects. The occasionally reported felt/neonatal side-effects include anemia, leukopenia, thrombocytopenia, decreased immunoglobulin levels, neonatal infection, and sepsis.

Corticosteroids

Prednisolone is the chief drug used for immunosuppression in post-transplant recipients. Initially used in higher doses in the first year, it is gradually tapered or completely discontinued. Maternal risks include the development of gestational hypertension, gestational diabetes mellitus, increased rates of premature rupture of membranes, and maternal and neonatal sepsis. Cleft lip and cleft palate can be seen with the usage of prednisone in the first trimester (US FDA category B). The fetal exposure to steroids is very low as the placenta metabolizes >90% of the maternal prednisone dose.

Mycophenolate Mofetil

It is a purine biosynthesis inhibitor that suppresses B- and T-cell function. It is US FDA category D medication and should be avoided. It is associated with spontaneous abortion (40%), cleft lip and cleft palate, microtia, absence of auditory canals neonatal anemia, and hypoplastic nails.

MATERNAL OUTCOMES

As per the current literature, there is no direct reported association between liver transplantation and maternal mortality. Gestational hypertension is commonly reported among liver transplant recipients between 2 and 43% and preeclampsia between 2 and 22%. The risk of development among liver transplant recipients is between 0 and 37.5%. Graft rejection rates during pregnancy vary from 0 to 20%. The rates of caesarean delivery are higher than vaginal delivery in liver transplant recipients (20–100%) attributed to increased rates of fetal distress due to gestational hypertension, preeclampsia, and gestational diabetes mellitus. The rates of vaginal delivery are variable (12.5–50%). Once the pregnancy is diagnosed, routine monitoring for the development of gestational hypertension and gestational diabetes mellitus should be undertaken.

FETAL OUTCOMES

The risk of spontaneous and missed abortions in liver transplant recipients (4.9–19%). The risk of stillbirths is 0–2%. Low birth weight <2,500 g has been observed in 4.8–57%. Fetal distress is seen in 10.3–40%. Overall congenital anomalies are uncommon and increased around 0–16.7%. Long-term follows up among babies born to mothers postliver transplant suggests that there is no abnormal physical development, adrenal or respiratory insufficiency, or lymphopenia or abnormal neurocognitive development.

BREASTFEEDING IN FEMALE LIVER TRANSPLANT RECIPIENTS ON IMMUNOSUPPRESSIVE THERAPY

Breastfeeding mothers on prednisone and other glucocorticoids can safely initiate breastfeeding, as advised by the American Academy of Pediatrics. Maternal tacrolimus therapy is compatible with breastfeeding. No adverse teratogenic effects are seen with maternal intake of azathioprine. Moreover, mothers should withhold breastfeeding the first few months after transplantation where the serum level of immunosuppressants is high.

CHAPTER 10

Multiple Choice Questions

1. **Which node is felt on the hepatic surface on percussion?**
   a. Resonant
   b. Tympanic
   c. Dull
   d. Hyperresonant

Ans. c. Dull

2. **Primary supports of the liver include all, except:**
   a. Coronary ligament
   b. Triangular ligament
   c. Duodenopancreatic complex
   d. Hepatic veins

Ans. c. Duodenopancreatic complex

3. **The two major surfaces of the liver are:**
   a. Anterior and posterior
   b. Anterosuperior and posteroinferior
   c. Anteroinferior and posterosuperior
   d. Dorsal and ventral

Ans. b. Anterosuperior and posteroinferior

4. **Falciform ligament of the liver is derived from:**
   a. Dorsal mesentery
   b. Ventral mesentery
   c. Ventral mesogastrium
   d. Dorsal mesogastrium

Ans. c. Ventral mesogastrium

5. **Which ligament connects the liver to the anterior abdominal wall?**
   a. Triangular ligament
   b. Falciform ligament
   c. Coronary ligament
   d. Ligamentum teres

Ans. d. Ligamentum teres

6. **Coronary ligaments attach the liver to:**
   a. Anterior abdominal wall
   b. Stomach
   c. Lesser omentum
   d. Diaphragm

Ans. d. Diaphragm

7. **Which structure contains the portal triad?**
   a. Greater omentum
   b. Lesser omentum
   c. Dorsal mesogastrium
   d. Ventral mesogastrium

Ans. b. Lesser omentum

8. Posteriorly the liver is related to all the organs, except:

a. Gallbladder
b. Pleura
c. IVC
d. Fundus of the stomach

Ans. b. Pleura

9. Which structure lies in the Cantlie's line?

a. Portal vein
b. Major hepatic vein
c. Major hepatic artery
d. Bile duct

Ans. b. Major hepatic vein

10. All of the following are true about portal vein, except:

a. The portal vein carries 80% of blood to the liver
b. The portal vein has valves
c. Portal vein acts as a blood reservoir
d. Normal portal venous pressure is 5–8 mm Hg

Ans. b. The portal vein has valves

11. Samples for the liver function tests are collected in which bulb?

a. EDTA bulb
b. Fluoride bulb
c. Plain bulb
d. Citrate bulb

Ans. c. Plain bulb

12. The upper limit of direct bilirubin:

a. 0.3 mg/dL
b. 0.5 mg/dL
c. 1 mg/dL
d. 10 mg/dL

Ans. a. 0.3 mg/dL

13. The lower bilirubin concentration with advanced gestational age is due to:

a. Decreased hepatic metabolism
b. Decreased RBC breakdown
c. Increased bilirubin excretion
d. Hemodilution

Ans. d. Hemodilution

14. Which enzyme is specifically elevated in liver cell damage?

a. Aspartate transaminase
b. Alanine transaminase
c. 5′-nucleotidase
d. Gamma-glutamyl transpeptidase

Ans. b. Alanine transaminase

15. ALT levels more than 1,000 IU/L are suggestive of all, except:

a. Intrahepatic cholestasis
b. Viral hepatitis
c. Ischemic liver disease
d. Toxin-induced hepatic damage

Ans. a. Intrahepatic cholestasis

16. Which is a false statement regarding alkaline phosphatase?

a. It is an isoenzyme
b. It is useful in differentiating between intrahepatic and extrahepatic causes
c. It is present in the liver, placenta, WBC
d. Levels increase as the gestational age advances

Ans. b. It is useful in differentiating between intrahepatic and extrahepatic causes

17. All the clotting factors are exclusively synthesized in the liver, except:

a. VII
b. VIII
c. IX
d. X

Ans. b. VIII

18. IHCP is most commonly seen during:

a. First trimester
b. Second trimester
c. Third trimester
d. Immediate postpartum

Ans. c. Third trimester

19. All of the following are false about IHCP, except:

a. Pruritus is the most important symptom
b. Pruritus is worsened during the evening
c. Pruritus is commonly seen over the back and abdomen
d. Pruritus is commonly seen over palms and soles

Ans. c. Pruritus is commonly seen over the back and abdomen

20. The upper limit of fasting bile acids for the diagnosis of IHCP is:

a. >5 micromole/L
b. >11 micromole>L
c. >18 micromole/L
d. >22 micromole/L

Ans. b. >11 micromole>L

21. Primary bile acids are:

a. Cholic and deoxycholic acid
b. Cholic and chenodeoxycholic acid
c. Glycocholic and taurocholic acid
d. Deoxycholic and deoxyglycocholic acid

Ans. b. Cholic and chenodeoxycholic acid

22. All of the following are involved in the management of IHCP, except:

a. Starting UDCA
b. Vitamin K to the neonate
c. Local emollients
d. Urgent caesarean section once the diagnosis is made

Ans. d. Urgent caesarean section once the diagnosis is made

23. Induction of labor in IHCP when the maternal and fetal parameters are normal is usually preferred at:

a. 34–35 weeks
b. 29–30 weeks
c. 37–38 weeks
d. 40–41 weeks

Ans. c. 37–38 weeks

24. All of the following are the fetal complications in IHCP, except:

a. MSAF
b. Prematurity
c. Fetal hyperbilirubinemia
d. Macrosomia and shoulder dystocia

Ans. d. Macrosomia and shoulder dystocia

25. A 30-year-old primigravida at 36 weeks of gestation presented with complaints of pruritus over palms and soles, jaundice, abdominal pain, vomiting, on investigation serum AST—102, ALT—110, fasting bile acids—24 micromole/L, most likely diagnosis is:

a. AFLP
b. Viral hepatitis
c. IHCP
d. HELLP syndrome

Ans. c. IHCP

26. Does acute fatty liver most commonly present in?

a. Second trimester
b. First trimester
c. Third trimester
d. 1 year after delivery

Ans. c. Third trimester

27. Incidence of AFLP in pregnancy:

a. 1 in 1,000
b. 1 in 10,000
c. 1 in 100
d. 1 in 100,000

Ans. b. 1 in 10,000

28. Dysfunction of which cellular organelle causes AFLP?

a. Mitochondria
b. Golgi body
c. Endoplasmic reticulum
d. Cytoplasmic membrane

Ans. a. Mitochondria

29. Which enzyme deficiency causes the accumulation of medium and long-chain fatty acids in the mitochondrial membrane?

a. Enoyl-CoA hydratase
b. 3-hydroxyacyl-CoA dehydrogenase
c. Thiokinase
d. Acetyl-CoA acetyltransferase

Ans. b. 3-hydroxyacyl-CoA dehydrogenase

30. All are risk factors for the development of AFLP in pregnancy, except:

a. Multigravida
b. Primigravida
c. Preeclampsia
d. Twin gestation

Ans. a. Multigravida

31. The most common sign of AFLP is:

a. Abdominal pain
b. Disseminated intravascular coagulation (DIC)
c. Jaundice
d. Itching over the palms and soles

Ans. c. Jaundice

32. Which criteria are used for the diagnosis of AFLP?

a. Edwards
b. Jefferson
c. Swansea
d. Donaldson

Ans. c. Swansea

33. All of the following are seen in AFLP, except:

a. Leukocytosis
b. Hyperglycemia
c. Hyperbilirubinemia
d. Coagulopathy

Ans. b. Hyperglycemia

34. The management of AFLP includes all, except:

a. Electrolyte correction
b. Fluid support
c. Emergency urgent caesarean section
d. Coagulopathy correction

Ans. c. Emergency urgent caesarean section

35. Risk of recurrence of ALFP in next pregnancy:

a. 5–10%
b. 1–2%
c. 70–80%
d. 25–35%

Ans. d. 25–35%

36. A 29-year-old primigravida, IVF conception presents to the emergency at 37 weeks of gestation with complaints of vomiting, jaundice, and headache. On examination, AST 500, ALT 423, platelets 80,000. A few hours later she complained of dizziness and altered sensorium. Most likely diagnosis in this case:

a. Intrahepatic cholestasis of pregnancy (IHCP)
b. AFLP
c. Viral hepatitis
d. Preeclampsia

Ans. d. Preeclampsia

37. The average incubation period of HAV is:

a. 30 days
b. 30 hours
c. 70 days
d. 100 days

Ans. a. 30 days

38. All are RNA viruses, except:

a. HAV
b. HBV
c. HCV
d. HEV

Ans. b. HBV

39. Severe acute hepatitis infection is caused by coinfection of:

a. HAV and HBV
b. HDV and HBV
c. HAV and HEV
d. HCV and HEV

Ans. b. HDV and HBV

40. High risk of progression to fulminant hepatitis in pregnancy is seen in:

a. HBV
b. HCV
c. HEV
d. HAV

Ans. c. HEV

41. False statement about HAV is:

a. Transmission is by the fecal-oral route
b. Infants born to HAV-infected mothers have high antibody and transaminase levels
c. No vertical transmission
d. IUGR and MSAF can be seen

Ans. b. Infants born to HAV-infected mothers have high antibody and transaminase levels

42. In pregnant women who are HBsAg positive, HBV DNA is done at:

a. 20 weeks
b. 24 weeks
c. 28 weeks
d. 36 weeks

Ans. c. 28 weeks

43. First-line treatment for HCV infection is:

a. Lamivudine
b. Tenofovir
c. Griseofulvin
d. Ribavirin

Ans. d. Ribavirin

44. Maternal mortality risk in HEV infection is:

a. 2%
b. 25%
c. 60%
d. 80%

Ans. b. 25%

45. The highest risk of cirrhosis and chronicity is seen with:

a. HBV
b. HCV
c. HDV
d. HEV

Ans. b. HCV

46. Infants born to HBsAg positive others should receive:
- a. Antiviral medications
- b. Only active immunization
- c. Only passive immunization
- d. Both active and passive immunization

Ans. d. Both active and passive immunization

47. Women with chronic liver disorders are unable to conceive due to:
- a. Hyperprolactinemia
- b. Gonadal atrophy
- c. Anovulation due to suppression of HPO axis
- d. Obesity and hyperandrogenism

Ans. c. Anovulation due to suppression of HPO axis

48. The highest risk of variceal bleeding is seen in which stage of labor?
- a. First stage
- b. Second stage
- c. Third stage
- d. Fourth stage

Ans. b. Second stage

49. Risk of maternal mortality with liver dysfunction is:
- a. 2%
- b. 18%
- c. 30%
- d. 45%

Ans. b. 18%

50. In patients with MELD score >10, the advice is:
- a. Early pregnancy registration
- b. Pregnancy is contraindicated
- c. Vaginal delivery preferred
- d. Emergency LSCS after 34 weeks

Ans. a. Early pregnancy registration

51. Prophylactic endoscopic ligation of varices is done in:
- a. First trimester
- b. Second trimester
- c. Third trimester
- d. Immediate postpartum

Ans. b. Second trimester

52. Which drug is avoided in chronic liver disease in pregnancy?
- a. Cephalosporins
- b. Beta-blockers
- c. Aspirin
- d. Digoxin

Ans. c. Aspirin

53. Hepatocellular carcinoma in pregnancy has a fulminant course due to:
- a. Decreased estrogen
- b. Increased Estrogen
- c. Shift to TH1 immunity
- d. Decreased progesterone

Ans. b. Increased Estrogen

54. Laboratory abnormalities seen in hepatocellular carcinoma include all, except:
a. Hypoalbuminemia
b. Decreased transaminases
c. Elevated clotting time
d. Hyperbilirubinemia

Ans. b. Decreased transaminases

55. The best possible management of HCC in pregnancy is:
a. Conservative management
b. Resection
c. Chemotherapy
d. Radiotherapy

Ans. b. Resection

56. The best prognosis in pregnancy is seen in which variety of HCC:
a. Scirrhous
b. Combined cholangiocarcinoma
c. Sarcomatoid
d. Fibrolamellar

Ans. d. Fibrolamellar

57. All of the following are risk factors for HCC, except:
a. HDV
b. HBV
c. Aflatoxins
d. Alcohol intake

Ans. a. HDV

58. Return of menstruation occurs after how many months post-liver transplantation:
a. 2 months
b. 3 months
c. 6 months
d. 12 months

Ans. b. 3 months

59. Post-transplantation conception should be delayed by:
a. 1 year
b. 2 years
c. 3 years
d. 5 years

Ans. a. 1 year

60. Cleft lip and cleft palate are the adverse effects seen with which immunosuppressants?
a. Corticosteroids
b. Mycophenolate mofetil
c. Azathioprine
d. Calcineurin

Ans. a. Corticosteroids

61. The most common complication in liver transplant recipients in pregnancy is:
a. Preeclampsia
b. Oligohydramnios
c. Postdatism
d. GDM

Ans. b. Oligohydramnios

62. A 21-year-old woman G3P2L2 at 34 weeks of gestation gives a history of vomiting and loose stools for 2 days, on examination she looks ill and icteric, laboratory markers ALT 1,200 AST 1,245, ALKP 700, most likely diagnosis:

a. HBV
b. HCV
c. HAV
d. HDV

Ans. c. HAV

63. A 32-year-old woman with twin gestation at 38 weeks of gestation presentedwithcomplaintsofheadacheandBPreadings140/100mmHg. CBC with peripheral smear suggestive of burr cells, schistocytes, and platelet count 1 lakh, AST 32 ALT 56, most likely diagnosis:

a. AFLP
b. Partial HELLP
c. Complete HELLP
d. IHCP

Ans. b. Partial HELLP

64. A 34-year-old pregnant woman presents to your OPD at 33 weeks of gestation with complaints of decreased fetal movements, NST-reactive, BPP 8/8. On investigation, AST 66 ALT 70, bile acids 15 μmol/L. All the following are done as a part of management, except:

a. Start UDCA
b. Weekly NST
c. Induction of labor
d. Antenatal steroids

Ans. c. Induction of labor

65. A woman presented for her first antenatal visit at 14 weeks of gestation, routine serological testing was conducted, serology report was suggestive HBsAg +, anti-HBS+, anti-HBC + IGM anti-HbC+, the likely diagnosis is:

a. Chronic infection
b. Acute infection
c. Immune due to natural infection
d. Immune due to vaccination

Ans. b. Acute infection

Index

Page numbers followed by *f* refer to figure, *fc* refer to flowchart, and *t* refer to table.